INTERVENTIONAL CARDIOLOGY CLINICS

www.interventional.theclinics.com

Editor-in-Chief

MARVIN H. ENG

Complex Coronary Interventions

October 2022 • Volume 11 • Number 4

Editor

Michael S. Lee

ELSEVIER

1600 John F. Kennedy Boulevard • Suite 1800 • Philadelphia, Pennsylvania, 19103-2899

http://www.theclinics.com

INTERVENTIONAL CARDIOLOGY CLINICS Volume 11, Number 4
October 2022 ISSN 2211-7458, ISBN-13: 978-0-323-98727-1

Editor: Joanna Collett
Developmental Editor: Arlene B. Campos

Interventional Cardiology Clinics (ISSN 2211-7458) is published quarterly by Elsevier Inc., 360 Park Avenue South, New York, NY 10010-1710. Months of issue are January, April, July, and October. Subscription prices are USD 209 per year for US individuals, USD 641 for US institutions, USD 100 per year for US students, USD 209 per year for Canadian individuals, USD 660 for Canadian institutions, USD 100 per year for Canadian students, USD 296 per year for international individuals, USD 660 for international institutions, and USD 150 per year for international students. To receive student/resident rate, orders must be accompanied by name of affiliated institution, date of term, and the *signature* of program/residency coordinator on institution letterhead. Orders will be billed at individual rate until proof of status is received. Foreign air speed delivery is included in all *Clinics* subscription prices. All prices are subject to change without notice. **POSTMASTER:** Send address changes to *Interventional Cardiology Clinics*, Elsevier Health Sciences Division, Subscription Customer Service, 3251 Riverport Lane, Maryland Heights, MO 63043. **Customer Service: Telephone: 1-800-654-2452** (U.S. and Canada); **1-314-447-8871** (outside U.S. and Canada). **Fax: 1-314-447-8029. E-mail: journalscustomerservice-usa@elsevier.com (for print support); journalsonlinesupport-usa@elsevier.com (for online support).**

Reprints. For copies of 100 or more of articles in this publication, please contact the Commercial Reprints Department, Elsevier Inc., 360 Park Avenue South, New York, NY 10010-1710. Tel.: 212-633-3874; Fax: 212-633-3820; E-mail: reprints@elsevier.com.

CONTRIBUTORS

EDITOR-IN-CHIEF

MARVIN H. ENG, MD
Structural Heart Program Medical Director, Structural Heart Disease Fellowship Director, Director of Cardiovascular Quality, Banner University Medical Center, Phoenix, Arizona, USA

EDITOR

MICHAEL S. LEE, MD, FACC, FSCAI
Associate Professor, Interventional Cardiology, UCLA Medical Center, Los Angeles, California, USA

AUTHORS

IBRAHIM AKIN, MD
First Department of Medicine, University Medical Centre Mannheim (UMM), Faculty of Medicine Mannheim, University of Heidelberg, European Center for AngioScience (ECAS), and DZHK (German Center for Cardiovascular Research) Partner Site Heidelberg/Mannheim, Mannheim, Germany

ZIAD A. ALI, MD, DPhil
St. Francis Hospital & Heart Center, Roslyn, New York, USA; Cardiovascular Research Foundation, Columbia University Irving Medical Center, New York, New York, USA

STEFAN BAUMANN, MD
First Department of Medicine, University Medical Centre Mannheim (UMM), Faculty of Medicine Mannheim, University of Heidelberg, European Center for AngioScience (ECAS), and DZHK (German Center for Cardiovascular Research) Partner Site Heidelberg/Mannheim, Mannheim, Germany

MICHAEL BEHNES, MD
First Department of Medicine, University Medical Centre Mannheim (UMM), Faculty of Medicine Mannheim, University of Heidelberg, European Center for AngioScience (ECAS), and DZHK (German Center for Cardiovascular Research) Partner Site Heidelberg/Mannheim, Mannheim, Germany

ADITYA S. BHARADWAJ, MD
Division of Cardiology, Department of Medicine, Loma Linda University Health, Loma Linda, California, USA

MARTIN BORGGREFE, MD
First Department of Medicine, University Medical Centre Mannheim (UMM), Faculty of Medicine Mannheim, University of Heidelberg, European Center for AngioScience (ECAS), and DZHK (German Center for Cardiovascular Research) Partner Site Heidelberg/Mannheim, Mannheim, Germany

PETER CANGIALOSI, MD
The Zena and Michael A. Wiener Cardiovascular Institute, Icahn School of Medicine at Mount Sinai, New York, New York, USA

DAVIDE CAO, MD
The Zena and Michael A. Wiener Cardiovascular Institute, Icahn School of Medicine at Mount Sinai, New York, New York, USA

SHAO-LIANG CHEN, MD
Nanjing First Hospital, Nanjing Medical University, Nanjing, China

SALVATORE DE ROSA, MD, PhD
Division of Cardiology, Department of Medical and Surgical Sciences, Research Center for Cardiovascular Diseases, "Magna Graecia" University, Catanzaro, Italy

ALOKE V. FINN, MD
CVPath Institute, Gaithersburg, Maryland,
USA; University of Maryland, School
of Medicine, Baltimore, Maryland,
USA

KEYVAN KARIMI GALOUGAHI, MD, PhD
St. Francis Hospital & Heart Center, Roslyn,
New York, USA

XIAO-FEI GAO, MD
Nanjing First Hospital, Nanjing Medical
University, Nanjing, China

ZHEN GE, MD
Nanjing First Hospital, Nanjing Medical
University, Nanjing, China

TOMMASO GORI, MD, PhD
Kardiologie I, Zentrum für Kardiologie,
University Medical Center Mainz, Deutsches
Zentrum für Herz und Kreislauf Forschung,
Standort Rhein-Main, Germany

CIRO INDOLFI, MD
Chief, Division of Cardiology, Department of
Medical and Surgical Sciences, Research
Center for Cardiovascular Diseases, "Magna
Graecia" University, Catanzaro, Italy;
Mediterranea Cardiocentro, Naples, Italy

ALLEN JEREMIAS, MD, MSc
St. Francis Hospital & Heart Center, Roslyn,
New York, USA; Cardiovascular Research
Foundation, New York, New York,
USA

KENJI KAWAI, MD
CVPath Institute, Gaithersburg, Maryland,
USA

DEAN J. KEREIAKES, MD, FACC, FSCAI
The Carl and Edyth Lindner Center for
Research and Education at The Christ
Hospital, Cincinnati, Ohio, USA

SEUNG-HYUN KIM, MD
First Department of Medicine, University
Medical Centre Mannheim (UMM), Faculty of
Medicine Mannheim, University of
Heidelberg, European Center for
AngioScience (ECAS), and DZHK (German
Center for Cardiovascular Research) Partner
Site Heidelberg/Mannheim, Mannheim,
Germany

JINHO LEE, MD
Department of Cardiology, Asan Medical
Center, University of Ulsan College of
Medicine, Songpa-gu, Seoul, Korea

MAMAS A. MAMAS, BM BCh, MA, DPhil, FRCP
Professor of Cardiology, Keele Cardiovascular
Research Group, Centre for Prognosis
Research, Institute for Primary Care and
Health Sciences, Keele University, United
Kingdom

ROXANA MEHRAN, MD
Professor, The Zena and Michael A. Wiener
Cardiovascular Institute, Icahn School of
Medicine at Mount Sinai, Center for
Interventional Cardiovascular Research and
Clinical Trials, New York, New York, USA

ANNALISA MONGIARDO, MD
Division of Cardiology, Department of
Medical and Surgical Sciences, "Magna
Graecia" University, Catanzaro, Italy

JOHNY NICOLAS, MD
The Zena and Michael A. Wiener
Cardiovascular Institute, Icahn School of
Medicine at Mount Sinai, New York, New
York, USA

DUK-WOO PARK, MD, PhD
Department of Cardiology, Asan Medical
Center, University of Ulsan College of
Medicine, Songpa-gu, Seoul, Korea

SEUNG-JUNG PARK, MD, PhD
Department of Cardiology, Asan Medical
Center, University of Ulsan College of
Medicine, Songpa-gu, Seoul, Korea

ALBERTO POLIMENI, MD, PhD
Division of Cardiology, Department of
Medical and Surgical Sciences, Research
Center for Cardiovascular Diseases, "Magna
Graecia" University, Catanzaro, Italy

ROBERT F. RILEY, MD
The Carl and Edyth Lindner Center for
Research and Education at The Christ
Hospital, Cincinnati, Ohio, USA

JOLANDA SABATINO, MD, PhD
Division of Cardiology, Department of
Medical and Surgical Sciences, Research

Center for Cardiovascular Diseases, "Magna Graecia" University, Catanzaro, Italy

ARNOLD H. SETO, MD, MPA, FSCAI, FACC
Long Beach Veterans Administration Medical Center, Long Beach, California, USA

EVAN SHLOFMITZ, DO
St. Francis Hospital & Heart Center, Roslyn, New York, USA

RICHARD A. SHLOFMITZ, MD
St. Francis Hospital & Heart Center, Roslyn, New York, USA

TIMOTHY D. SMITH, MD
The Carl and Edyth Lindner Center for Research and Education at The Christ Hospital, Cincinnati, Ohio, USA

SABATO SORRENTINO, MD, PhD
Division of Cardiology, Department of Medical and Surgical Sciences, Research Center for Cardiovascular Diseases, "Magna Graecia" University, Catanzaro, Italy

CARMEN SPACCAROTELLA, MD
Division of Cardiology, Department of Medical and Surgical Sciences, Research Center for Cardiovascular Diseases, "Magna Graecia" University, Catanzaro, Italy

ALESSANDRO SPIRITO, MD
The Zena and Michael A. Wiener Cardiovascular Institute, Icahn School of Medicine at Mount Sinai, New York, New York, USA

DAVID M. TEHRANI, MD, MS
University of California, Los Angeles, Los Angeles, California, USA

SUSAN V. THOMAS, MPH
St. Francis Hospital & Heart Center, Roslyn, New York, USA

RENU VIRMANI, MD
CVPath Institute, Gaithersburg, Maryland, USA

JUN-JIE ZHAN, MD, PhD
Nanjing First Hospital, Nanjing Medical University, Nanjing, China

CONTENTS

Traditionally, the treatment of left main coronary artery disease is recommended coronary artery bypass grafting because of its superior long-term outcomes compared with medical treatment and plain old balloon angioplasty. However, improvement of percutaneous coronary intervention technique and introduction of drug-eluting stent led to change of treatment strategy of left main coronary artery disease through cumulative data for revascularization that based on clinical evidence.

Moderate-severe calcification increases procedural complications and impairs long-term prognosis post-PCI. Intravascular imaging (particularly optical coherence tomography [OCT]) is useful in guiding the treatment of calcified lesions. Weighted sum of calcium length, arc, and thickness on OCT can predict adequate stent expansion, identifying when atherectomy is required. With intravascular imaging guidance, various techniques alone or in combination may be used in an algorithmic fashion to modify calcified lesions. Calcium fracture by balloon angioplasty, cutting/scoring balloons, intravascular lithotripsy (IVL), atherectomy devices, or Excimer laser improves stent expansion. Intravascular imaging is essential in the treatment of in-stent restenosis when luminal and/or abluminal peri-strut calcium is present.

Even though saphenous vein grafts (SVGs) are the most commonly used surgical conduits, their long-term patency is limited by accelerated atherosclerosis often resulting in acute coronary syndrome or asymptomatic occlusion. SVG intervention is associated with 2 significant challenges: a significant risk of distal embolization with resultant periprocedural myocardial infarction in the short-term and restenosis in the long-term. Several individual trials have compared bare metal stents with drug-eluting stents for SVG intervention. This review article discusses the pathophysiology of SVG lesions, indications for SVG intervention, and the challenges encountered, and also technical considerations for SVG intervention and the supporting evidence.

Intravascular lithotripsy (IVL) uses acoustic shock waves in a balloon-based delivery system to modify severely calcified atherosclerotic coronary vascular lesions in preparation for stent implantation. IVL results in circumferential and longitudinal calcium fracture, which improves transmural vessel compliance and facilitates subsequent stent expansion without requiring high-pressure balloon dilation. Clinical trials have demonstrated IVL to be safe (low rates of major adverse cardiac events in hospital and to 1 year; low rates of severe angiographic complications), effective (high rates of procedural success), and easy to use (little or no learning curve) when applied in the treatment of severely calcified coronary arteries.

Percutaneous coronary intervention (PCI) with drug-eluting stent (DES) for the treatment of coronary bifurcation lesions (CBLs) is still technically demanding, mainly because of higher rates of both acute and chronic complication as compared with non-CBLs. Although provisional stenting (PS) is considered as the preferred strategy for most of the CBLs, a systematic two-stent technique (double kissing [DK] crush) should be considered in patients with complex left main (LM)-CBLs or non–LM-CBLs stratified by the DEFINITION criteria. Intracoronary imaging and/or physiologic evaluation should be used to optimize CBLs intervention. PCI with DES for the treatment of CBLs is technically demanding, mainly because of higher rates of both acute and chronic complication as compared with non-CBLs. PS is a default strategy for most of the CBLs. Double kissing (DK) crush is associated with better clinical outcomes compared with PS in patients with complex LM-CBLs or non–LM-CBLs stratified by the DEFINITION criteria. Intracoronary imaging and/or physiologic evaluation are useful tools to guide the treatment of CBLs. The use of drug-coated balloons in CBLs needs further data to support the clinical benefits.

Antithrombotic therapy is the cornerstone of secondary cardiovascular prevention after percutaneous coronary intervention (PCI). Improvements in drug-eluting stent (DES) design and materials over the last 2 decades have prompted the development of new antithrombotic strategies. Current guidelines recommend to tailor dual antiplatelet therapy (DAPT) according to clinical presentation and individual ischemic and bleeding risk. Given the growing number of complex PCI procedures performed nowadays, it is a priority to define the optimal antithrombotic treatment in this challenging patient subset. In this review article, we sought to summarize and discuss the current evidence on antiplatelet therapy in patients undergoing complex PCI.

In-stent restenosis (ISR) remains a potential complication after percutaneous coronary intervention, even in the era of drug-eluting stents, and its treatment remains suboptimal. Neoatherosclerosis is an important component of the pathology of ISR and is accelerated in drug-eluting stents compared with bare-metal stents. Coronary angiography is the gold standard for evaluating the morphology of ISR, although computed tomography angiography is emerging as an alternative noninvasive modality to evaluate the presence of ISR. Drug-coated balloons and stent reimplantation are the current mainstays of treatment for ISR, and the choice of treatment should be based on clinical background and lesion morphology.

> Coronary complications are increasingly rare but remain fatal if not managed promptly and effectively. We review the incidence, management, and prevention of the most serious coronary complications including acute vessel closure from dissection, no-reflow, thrombosis, and air embolism as well as mechanical complications including perforation, stent dislodgment, and atherectomy burr entrapment.

> The evolution of percutaneous coronary intervention (PCI) enables a complete revascularization of complex coronary lesions. However, simultaneously, patients are presenting nowadays with higher rates of comorbidities, which may lead to a lower physiologic tolerance for complex PCI. To avoid hemodynamic instability during PCI and achieve safe complete revascularization, protected PCI using mechanical circulatory support devices has been developed. However, which patients would benefit from the protected PCI is still in debate. Hence, this review provides practical approaches for the selection of patients by outlining current clinical data assessing utility of protected PCI in high-risk patients.

> Since their introduction in clinical practice in 1986, different types of coronary stents have been developed and become available for the treatment of coronary artery disease. Stent thrombosis (ST) is an uncommon but harmful complication after percutaneous coronary implantation, with a high occurrence of acute myocardial infarction and risk of mortality. Among several procedural and clinical predictors, the type of coronary stent is a strong determinant of ST. This article reviews the available evidence on the most used coronary stent types in the modern era and the related risk of ST.

COMPLEX CORONARY INTERVENTIONS

SERIES OF RELATED INTEREST

Cardiology Clinics
Cardiac Electrophysiology Clinics
Heart Failure Clinics

THE CLINICS ARE NOW AVAILABLE ONLINE!

Access your subscription at:
www.theclinics.com

FOREWORD

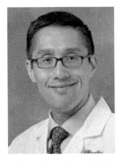

Marvin H. Eng, MD
Consulting Editor

We are pleased to introduce this issue of *Interventional Cardiology Clinics* discussing the updates in percutaneous coronary intervention (PCI). While there is some overlap with coronary chronic total occlusion PCI, the subject of complex PCI encompasses treatment of a broader patient and lesion substrate generalizable to nearly all interventionalists. Despite the rapid expansion of other subdisciplines in interventional cardiology (ie, structural, peripheral), coronary artery disease treatment remains the core role of interventional cardiologists.

The improvements in PCI have grown in several directions: technology, technique, and pharmacology. Recent analysis from a real-world registry reflects that a recent increase in PCI volume has been observed at least in some parts of the United States.[1] Several national registries have documented increasing patient complexity and risk profiles for PCI,[2,3] meaning that PCI volume is durable but becoming more challenging. Whether one is treating obstinate, calcified lesions or high-risk bypass grafts, refined tools and techniques are needed for optimizing PCI results. Bifurcation PCI, including left main PCI, is a common dilemma that may combine calcification, tortuosity, angulation, and elevated myocardial jeopardy. Technical advances in these advanced lesion subsets and optimized pharmacology are the keys to improving outcomes. As usual, no lessons about complex PCI are complete without discussing complications management.

This issue of *Interventional Cardiology Clinics* has been edited by Dr Michael Lee, a veteran operator and paragon of excellence in PCI. We congratulate Dr Lee for assembling a comprehensive update of PCI. Readership should find this issue to be a practical and worthwhile investment in their continuing growth.

Marvin H. Eng, MD
Banner University Medical Center
1111 East McDowell Road
Phoenix, AZ 85006, USA

E-mail address:
engm@email.arizona.edu

REFERENCES

1. Kataruka A, Maynard CC, Kearney KE, et al. Temporal trends in percutaneous coronary intervention and coronary artery bypass grafting: insights from the Washington Cardiac Care Outcomes Assessment Program. J Am Heart Assoc 2020;9:e015317.
2. Waldo SW, Gokhale M, O'Donnell CI, et al. Temporal trends in coronary angiography and percutaneous coronary intervention: insights from the VA Clinical Assessment, Reporting, and Tracking Program. JACC Cardiovasc Interv 2018;11:879–88.
3. Vora AN, Dai D, Gurm H, et al. Temporal trends in the risk profile of patients undergoing outpatient percutaneous coronary intervention. Circ Cardiovasc Interv 2016;9:e003070.

PREFACE

Disruptive Innovation to the Field of Interventional Cardiology

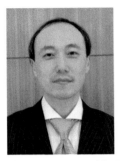

Michael S. Lee, MD, FACC, FSCAI
Editor

It is my pleasure and honor to introduce the latest issue of "Complex Coronary Intervention" in *Interventional Cardiology Clinics*. It has been 6 years since the last issue of "Complex Coronary Intervention" was published. This issue includes some of the most influential interventional cardiologists of all time, including Dr Seung-Jung Park, who is widely considered the father of left main percutaneous coronary intervention (PCI). His pioneering work in left main disease pushed the envelope to treat lesions that were previously considered taboo. Under his leadership, Dr Park and the Asan Medical Center in Seoul, South Korea have contributed more data than any other group, and the Asan Medical Center is the epicenter of left main PCI. Dr Park's relentless pursuit of scientific data and mastery of left main PCI technique will be one of the hallmarks of his legacy. His conference, TCT Asia Pacific, just had its 27th scientific session in 2022.

The author of the article on calcium modification is Dr Richard Shlofmitz, who is widely considered the foremost expert and has the most experience in the treatment of severely calcified coronary artery disease. As one of the most prolific operators in the world who keeps a schedule that is unparalleled to anyone else, his strategy of optimizing PCI with intravascular imaging and plaque modification has set the benchmark for PCI. His leadership has attracted some of the most well-recognized names in coronary physiology and intravascular imaging to St. Francis Hospital in Roslyn, New York. Dr Shlofmitz is now joined by his son, Dr Evan Shlofmitz, a rising star and future leader in our field. Their conference, Optimizing PCI: Intravascular Imaging and Coronary Physiology, just had its 8th annual meeting in 2022.

One of the new technologies that was introduced is intravascular lithotripsy, which is a "disruptive" innovation to the field of interventional cardiology. Using the same principles of treating nephrolithiasis, lithotripsy can fracture severe coronary artery calcification, which facilitates stent delivery and optimal stent expansion. Dr Dean Kereiakes, a legendary interventionist and Principal Investigator of the DISRUPT CAD III trial, provides a comprehensive overview of this novel technology, which simplifies the treatment of this complex disease subset.

Optimal antiplatelet therapy is a rapidly evolving topic. One of the most influential experts, Dr Roxana Mehran, and her group at Mt. Sinai Hospital in New York, New York, summarizes the current treatment paradigm for antiplatelet therapy, including deescalation for those who are at high risk for bleeding complications.

Under his leadership, Dr Shao-Liang Chen and his group at Nanjing First Hospital in Nanjing, China have published the DKCRUSH series of clinical trials. The double-kissing (DK) crush technique

Intervent Cardiol Clin 11 (2022) xiii–xiv
https://doi.org/10.1016/j.iccl.2022.07.003
2211-7458/22/© 2022 Published by Elsevier Inc.

is widely used to treat complex bifurcation disease in many geographies. Data continue to demonstrate that this technique is safe and effective for this complex lesion subset.

I am indebted to all the authors who dedicated their valuable time out of their busy practices to contribute to this issue of *Interventional Cardiology Clinics*. This issue truly represents an international perspective of interventional cardiology, which includes authors from Asia, Europe, and North America. I look forward to the next issue, where new technology, techniques, and optimization of treatment paradigms will improve patient outcomes. Until then, I hope you enjoy our latest issue.

Michael S. Lee, MD, FACC, FSCAI
Interventional Cardiology
UCLA Medical Center
100 Medical Plaza, Suite 630
Los Angeles, CA 90095, USA

E-mail address:
michaelsblee@gmail.com

Left Main Disease

Jinho Lee, MD[a], Duk-Woo Park, MD, PhD[a], Seung-Jung Park, MD, PhD[a],*

KEYWORDS

- Left main coronary artery disease • Percutaneous coronary intervention
- Coronary artery bypass surgery • Revascularization strategy

KEY POINTS

- For the treatment of left main coronary artery (LMCA) disease, percutaneous coronary intervention (PCI) is an alternative therapeutic option, especially in patients with an SYNTAX score ≤32, given the improvement of PCI technologies and refined techniques for the treatment of distal bifurcation disease.
- The current strategy for revascularization of LMCA disease requires a multidisciplinary Heart Team approach and extensive patient counseling to obtain informed consent.
- Evaluation of lesion severity and stent optimization with physiologic assessment and intravascular imaging, respectively, can improve clinical outcomes following PCI for LMCA disease.

Introduction

Left main coronary artery (LMCA) disease, which is defined as ≥50% diameter stenosis by visual estimation, is found in 4% to 7% of patients who underwent coronary angiography. Because the LMCA supplies a major portion of the myocardium, LMCA disease portends a poor prognosis when compared with other types of coronary artery disease (CAD).[1] Therefore, the 2014 American College of Cardiology (ACC)/American Heart Association (AHA) guidelines strongly recommended that patients with an LMCA stenosis of ≥50% undergo revascularization.[2] Since the 1970s, coronary artery bypass grafting (CABG) has been regarded as the standard of care for unprotected LMCA disease because it has superior long-term outcomes compared with medical treatment and plain old balloon angioplasty.[3,4] However, percutaneous coronary intervention (PCI) with drug-eluting stents (DES) represents a significant improvement compared with the era of balloon angioplasty for the treatment of severe LMCA disease. Furthermore, refinements in revascularization techniques and antithrombotic therapy are associated with low rates of ischemic complications.[5] Recently, several randomized controlled trials (RCTs) comparing PCI and CABG were published. This article reviews the current clinical evidence based on cumulative data for revascularization for LMCA disease, physiologic and anatomic lesion assessment, and risk stratification to optimize decision-making.

Treatment Strategies for LMCA Disease

Treatment guidelines for LMCA disease

Currently, the 2 guidelines for the optimal treatment strategy for LMCA disease are based on several registry studies and RCTs. Guidelines from the European Society of Cardiology and the ACC/AHA state that CABG surgery is the standard of care for LMCA disease with a class I indication.[2,6–8] However, the 2 guidelines provided slightly different recommendations for PCI in LMCA disease. The 2014 ESC guidelines state that PCI for LMCA disease with an intermediate Synergy Between Percutaneous Coronary Intervention with TAXUS and Cardiac Surgery (SYNTAX) score (22–32) has a class IIa indication with a level of evidence B. In the case of LMCA disease with more complexity (SYNTAX

a Department of Cardiology, Asan Medical Center, University of Ulsan College of Medicine, 88, Olympic-ro 43-gil, Songpa-gu, Seoul 05505, Korea
* Corresponding author.
E-mail addresses: dwpark@amc.seoul.kr (D.-W.P.); sjpark@amc.seoul.kr (S.-J.P.)

Intervent Cardiol Clin 11 (2022) 359–371
https://doi.org/10.1016/j.iccl.2022.02.006
2211-7458/22/© 2022 Elsevier Inc. All rights reserved.

score >32), the guidelines state that there is a class III indication with a level of evidence B. After the publication of several RCTs and observational studies that showed noninferiority with PCI compared with CABG for LMCA disease, the updated 2018 ESC guidelines elevated the level of evidence from B to A for PCI in LMCA disease with an intermediate SYNTAX score (22–32). In contrast, the 2014 ACC/AHA guidelines provide a class IIa indication with a level of evidence B for PCI in patients with LMCA and low anatomic risk (SYNTAX score < 22 or disease location at the ostial or trunk of the LMCA), a class IIb indication for those with intermediate anatomic risk (SYNTAX score 22–32), and a class IIIb indication for patients with unfavorable anatomy (SYNTAX score ≥33). The updated 2021 ACC/AHA guidelines elevated the class of recommendation of PCI in LMCA disease with medium anatomic risk from IIb to IIa. In LMCA disease with low-to-mediate anatomic complexity, PCI is reasonable to improve survival when PCI can provide equivalent revascularization to that possible with CABG[8] (Table 1).

Clinical evidence for LMCA disease
Advancements in stent technology, especially with the introduction of second-generation DES, which are safer and more efficacious compared with first-generation DES, and refinements in stent technique have resulted in improved clinical outcomes. Meta-analyses from 6 RCTs also suggest comparable results with PCI and CABG for the treatment of LMCA disease (Table 2).

Randomized controlled trials.
The first RCT comparing the safety and efficacy of CABG and PCI for patients with LMCA disease was the LE MANS trial,[9] in which 105 patients with LMCA stenosis were randomized to PCI or CABG. The primary end point was the change in the left ventricular ejection fraction (LVEF) 12 months after revascularization. The secondary end points were major adverse events (MAE) and major adverse cardiac and cerebrovascular events (MACCE) at 30 days and 1 year. At 1-year follow-up, the PCI group reported a significant increase in LVEF compared with the CABG group (3.3 ± 6.7% vs 0.5 ± 0.8%; P = .047) as well as a lower 30-day risk of MAE (P < .006) and MACCE (P = .03), and a shorter length of hospitalization (P = .0007).

The SYNTAX trial[10] randomized 1800 patients with de novo 3-vessel disease and/or LMCA disease to PCI with paclitaxel-eluting stents and CABG. In the subgroup of 705 patients with

LMCA disease, the primary end point of MACCE at 1 year was similar in the CABG and PCI groups (13.7% vs 15.8%; P = .44). In the secondary outcomes, stroke at 1 year was significantly higher in the CABG group (2.7% vs 0.3%; P = .009). However, repeat revascularization at 1 year was significantly higher in the PCI group (6.5% vs 11.8%; P = .02).

The Premier of Randomized Comparison of Bypass Surgery versus Angioplasty Using Sirolimus-Eluting Stent in Patients with Left Main Coronary Artery Disease (PRECOMBAT) trial enrolled 600 patients with LMCA disease who were randomized to CABG or PCI with sirolimus-eluting stents.[11] PCI with sirolimus-eluting stents was noninferior to CABG with respect to MACCE at 1 year (8.7% vs 6.7%, P = .01 for noninferiority). MACCE at 2 years was not significantly different between PCI and CABG (12.2% vs 8.1%; hazard ratio [HR] with PCI, 1.50; 95% confidence interval [CI], 0.90–2.52; P = .12).

In the randomized comparison of PCI with sirolimus-eluting stents versus CABG for the LMCA stenosis trial,[12] 201 patients with LMCA disease were randomized to PCI with sirolimus-eluting stent or CABG using predominantly arterial grafts. PCI was noninferior to CABG with respect to the primary end point of major adverse cardiovascular event (MACE) at 12-month follow-up (19.0% vs 13.9%, P = .19 for noninferiority). The rate of death and myocardial infarction (MI) was comparable between CABG and PCI (7.9% vs 5.0%, P < .001 for noninferiority). However, repeat revascularization was inferior in the PCI group compared with the CABG group (14.0% vs 5.9%, P = .35 for noninferiority).

These 4 RCTs comparing PCI using early-generation DES versus CABG for LMCA disease demonstrated similar clinical outcomes at short-term follow-up. The 10-year outcomes of the LE MANS trial[13] showed that patients who underwent PCI had a numerically higher LVEF and had no significant differences in mortality and MACCE. In the PRECOMBAT trial,[14] the incidence of MACCE was not significantly different between the PCI and CABG groups at extended follow-up (29.8% vs 24.7%). Similarly, the composite of death, MI, or stroke and all-cause mortality were not significantly different between the 2 groups. The 5-year outcomes of the left main subgroup of the SYNTAX trial[15] demonstrated no difference in overall MACCE between the PCI and CABG groups. Consistent with previous studies, the PCI group had a lower rate of stroke and a higher rate of repeat revascularization.

Table 1 Current guidelines of PCI for LMCA disease		
Guidelines	**Class of Recommendation**	**Level of Evidence**
2018 ESC/EACTS[7]	I—LMCA with an SYNTAX score ≤ 22 IIa—LMCA with an SYNTAX score 23–32 III—LMCA with an SYNTAX score ≥ 33	A
2014 ACC/AHA[2]	IIa—For SIHD patients when both of the following are present: • Anatomic conditions associated with a low risk of PCI procedural complications and a high likelihood of good long-term outcomes (eg, a low SYNTAX score of ≤ 22, ostial or trunk left main CAD) • Clinical characteristics that predict a significantly increased risk of adverse surgical outcomes (eg, STS-predicted risk of operative mortality ≥ 5%)	B
	IIb—For SIHD when both of the following are present: • Anatomic conditions associated with a low to intermediate risk of PCI procedural complications and an intermediate to high likelihood of good long-term outcomes (eg, low-intermediate SYNTAX score of < 33, bifurcation left main CAD) • Clinical characteristics that predict an increased risk of adverse surgical outcomes (eg, moderate-severe COPD, disability from prior stroke, or prior cardiac surgery; STS-predicted operative mortality >2%)	B
	III—For SIHD in patients (vs performing CABG) with unfavorable anatomy for PCI and who are good candidates for CABG	B
2021 ACC/AHA[8]	IIa—In selected patients with SIHD and significant left main stenosis for whom PCI can provide equivalent revascularization to that possible with CABG, PCI is reasonable to improve survival	B

Abbreviations: COPD, chronic obstructive pulmonary disease; SIHD, stable ischemic heart disease; STS, Society of Thoracic Surgeons.

The current ACC/AHA and ESC guidelines were based on the results of these 4 RCTs. However, the limitations of these RCTs were that they were underpowered because of the small sample size and the wide noninferiority margin. Furthermore, first-generation DES, which have higher rates of stent thrombosis and repeat revascularization, were used in these 4 RCTs. Subsequently, 2 landmark RCTs were conducted with more contemporary DES.

In the Everolimus Eluting Stents or Bypass Surgery for Left Main Coronary Artery Disease (EXCEL) trial,[16] 1905 patients with LMCA disease and low or intermediate anatomic complexity (SYNTAX score ≤32) were randomized to PCI with fluoropolymer-based cobalt-chromium everolimus-eluting stents (948 patients) or CABG (957 patients). PCI was noninferior to CABG with respect to the primary end point event of MACE at 3 years (15.4% vs 14.7%; $P = .02$ for noninferiority). However, PCI was superior to CABG with respect to the secondary end point event of death, stroke, or MI at 30 days (4.9% vs 7.9%; $P < .001$ for noninferiority, $P = .008$ for superiority). PCI was also noninferior with respect to the composite of death, MI, stroke, and ischemia-driven revascularization at 3 years (23.1% vs 19.1%). The 5-year follow-up[17] also demonstrated no significant difference in MACE between the PCI and CABG groups (22% vs 19.2%; $P = .13$). Although cardiovascular death and MI were not significantly different between the PCI and CABG groups (5.0% vs 4.5%, 10.6% vs 9.1%, respectively), all-cause death was higher in the PCI group compared with the CABG group (13.9% vs 9.9%).

Table 2
Randomized controlled trials of PCI versus CABG for LMCA disease

	Recruitment Period	N (PCI/CABG)	Diabetes (%)	Bifurcation (%)	SYNTAX Score, (Mean)	Stent Type	Primary End Point	Follow-Up (y)	Key Findings
LE MANS[9,13]	2001–2004	52/53	18	58	Not reported	BMS and DES	Improvement of LVEF	10	Improvement LVEF in PCI at 10 y
Boudriot et al.[12]	2003–2009	100/101	36	72	23	DP-SES	Death, MI, stroke, or RR	1	PCI inferior to CABG at 1 y
PRECOMBAT[11,14]	2004–2009	300/300	32	64	25	DP-SES	Death, MI, stroke, or TVR	10	PCI noninferior to CABG at 1, 5, and 10 y
SYNTAX[10,15]	2005–2007	357/348	25	61	30	DP-PES	Death, MI, stroke, or RR	5	PCI comparable to CABG at 1 and 5 y
EXCEL[16,17]	2010–2014	948/957	5	81	21	DP-EES	Death, MI, or stroke	5	PCI noninferior to CABG at 3 and 5 y
NOBLE[18,19]	2008–2015	592/592	5	81	22	BP-BES and DP-SES	Death, nonprocedural MI, stroke, or RR	5	PCI was inferior to CABG at 5 y

Abbreviations: BMS, bare-metal stent; BP-BES, biodegradable-polymer biolimus-eluting stent; DP-EES, durable-polymer everolimus-eluting stent; DP-PES, durable-polymer paclitaxel-eluting stent; DP-SES, durable-polymer sirolimus-eluting stent; LVEF, left ventricular ejection fraction; MI, myocardial infarction; RR, repeat revascularization; TVR, target vessel revascularization.

In the Nordic-Baltic-British left main revascularization (NOBLE) trial,[18] 1201 patients with LMCA disease were randomly assigned to PCI (n = 598) or CABG (n = 603). The primary end point of MACCE at 5 years was lower in the CABG group compared with PCI (19% vs 29%, P = .0066). The secondary end points of nonprocedural MI and any revascularization were higher in the PCI group compared with the CABG group (16% vs 10%; P = .004, 5% vs 2%; P = .073, respectively). All-cause mortality at 5-year was not significantly different between the PCI and CABG groups (28% vs 19%; P = .77). The updated 5-year clinical outcomes of the NOBLE trial[19] also demonstrated a lower MACCE rate with CABG (19% vs 28%; P = .0002) and similar all-cause mortality in the 2 groups (9% vs 9%). However, the rates of nonprocedural MI and repeat revascularization were lower in the CABG group (3% vs 8%; P = .0002, 10% vs 17%; P = .0009, respectively).

The discordant results from the EXCEL and NOBLE trials may be due to several factors including different study designs, patient assessment, patient characteristics, and definition of MI. Longer-term follow-up can help determine the optimal revascularization strategy for LMCA disease.

Meta-analysis. Various meta-analyses have compared the safety and efficacy of PCI with bare-metal stent or DES and CABG for LMCA disease.[20,21] Recent meta-analyses have included with results of the EXCEL and NOBLE trials, which used second-generation DES.

In the meta-analysis by Giacoppo and colleagues[22], which included 4 RCTs (SYNTAX, PRECOMBAT, EXCEL, and NOBLE), the primary end point of the composite of all-cause death, MI, or stroke at 3 to 5 years showed no significant difference between the PCI and CABG groups (16.9% vs 18.3%). Upadhaya and colleagues performed a meta-analysis of 5 RCTs with 4595 patients with LMCA. The primary end point of MACCE (death, MI, stroke, or repeat revascularization) was higher in the PCI group compared with the CABG group (odds ratio [OR] 1.36; 95% CI, 1.18–1.58; P < .0001), which was driven by a higher rate of repeat revascularization (OR 1.85; 95% CI, 1.53–2.23; P < .00001). However, the rate of MI, stroke, or cardiac and all-cause mortality were not significantly different between the 2 groups.[23] Ahmad and colleagues performed a meta-analysis of 5 RCTs (NOBLE, SYNTAX, EXCEL, PRECOMBAT, Boudriot and colleagues) including the 10-year outcomes of the SYNTAX

trial. The overall long-term mortality was similar in the PCI with DES group compared with the CABG group (relative risk [RR] 1.03; 95% CI, 0.79–1.34; P = .817), as was the composite of cardiac death, stroke, or MI.[24] Kuno and colleagues performed a meta-analysis of 4 RCTs that had at least 5-year follow-up. All-cause death was similar in both groups (HR 1.13; 95% CI, 0.88–1.44; P = .34). The risk of cardiovascular death, stroke, and MI was not significantly different between the 2 groups. However, repeat revascularization was significantly higher in the PCI group compared with the CABG group (HR 1.80; 95% CI, 1.52–2.13; P < .01).[25]

Based on the RCTs and meta-analyses, the overall results suggest a comparable risk for mortality and the composite of death, MI, or stroke at long-term follow-up. The CABG group had higher rates of procedural MI and stroke compared with the PCI group, whereas the risk of spontaneous MI and repeat revascularization was higher in the PCI group.

Special consideration

Risk stratification. Various scoring systems are available to risk stratify patients with LMCA disease to help clinicians determine the ideal revascularization strategy. The SYNTAX score, which is based on the anatomic complexity of the coronary artery lesions on angiography, can guide the clinical decision-making between CABG and PCI.[26] The high SYNTAX score group has more complex CAD, which makes achieving complete revascularization with PCI more difficult. CABG provided superior outcomes in this group compared with PCI.[27,28] Although long-term mortality was not significantly different between PCI and CABG when stratified by the SYNTAX score, MACCE was higher in the PCI group in the high SYNTAX score group.[29] Other scoring tools such as the EuroSCORE, STS score, and ACEF score incorporate baseline clinical characteristics and comorbidities, which may provide further insight into the surgical risk and help decision-making as CABG is generally less affected by the coronary artery complexity.[30] The SYNTAX score II was developed to incorporate both the clinical characteristics and the complexity of the coronary artery.[31] The SYNTAX score II contains 8 predictors, which include the anatomic SYNTAX score and patient clinical characteristics such as age, creatinine clearance, LVEF, presence of LMCA disease, peripheral vascular disease, female sex, and chronic obstructive pulmonary disease. At cross-validation, the newly developed SYNTAX score

II, called the SYNTAX Score II 2020, was able to predict 10-year death and 5-year MACE.[32]

Patient with diabetes. Diabetes is an important predictor of long-term outcomes after coronary revascularization because these patients have more complex CAD that is often characterized by long, diffuse lesions and higher rates of restenosis after PCI compared with nondiabetic patients. The FREEDOM (Comparison of Two Treatments for Multivessel Coronary Artery Disease in Individuals with Diabetes) trial demonstrated that CABG was superior to PCI in terms of reducing death and MI in diabetic patients and multivessel CAD.[33] On the contrary, the impact of diabetes in LMCA disease is less clearly defined[34] (Fig. 1). Subgroup analysis of diabetic patients in the EXCEL trial showed comparable clinical outcomes with PCI and CABG.[35] The MAIN-COMPARE (Revascularization for Unprotected Left Main Coronary Artery Stenosis: Comparison of Percutaneous Coronary Angioplasty vs Surgical Revascularization) registry reported no significant difference in 10-year clinical outcomes including all-cause mortality in diabetic patients between the PCI and CABG groups.[36] Therefore, unlike in multivessel CAD, the impact of diabetes in guiding the optimal revascularization strategy for LMCA disease has a limited role. Henceforth, PCI appears to be a reasonable option in diabetic patients with LMCA disease and low or intermediate anatomic complexity.

Patients with heart failure with reduced ejection fraction. The LMCA supplies blood flow to a large portion of the myocardium. Therefore, patients with advanced LMCA disease may have reduced LVEF due to myocardial ischemia. Surgical revascularization provided a survival benefit compared with medical therapy for these patients.[37] Although no RCTs have been performed, a meta-analysis including 16 observational studies demonstrated that the CABG group had a lower mortality compared with the PCI group in patients with CAD and LVEF ≤40% (HR 0.82; 95% CI, 0.75–0.90; $P < .001$).[38] In patients with LMCA disease and moderate to severe reduction in LVEF, there was a trend toward a lower risk of the composite outcome of death, MI, or stroke with CABG compared with PCI.[39] However, the difference in the event rate decreased if PCI resulted in complete revascularization. Therefore, multiple variables such as surgical risk and the likelihood of achieving complete revascularization with PCI should be considered when evaluating the ideal revascularization strategy for patients with LMCA disease and reduced LVEF.

Heart Team approach

When evaluating a patient with LMCA disease for surgical or percutaneous revascularization, various factors should be considered including the patient's age, clinical condition, likelihood of achieving complete revascularization, and complexity of the coronary anatomy. The current guidelines recommend a Heart Team approach, which involves a multidisciplinary approach with a cardiologist and cardiac surgeon during the decision-making and informed consent process to determine the most appropriate treatment of each individual patient.[5,8,40]

Evaluation of Left Main Coronary Artery Disease

Coronary angiography is considered the gold standard for the evaluation of CAD. However, the ability to assess the extent of LMCA disease is limited because of the high prevalence of bifurcation disease, lesion angulation, and the lack of a reference segment.[41] These limitations can lead to the inability to determine the degree of functional impairment caused by LMCA disease. In one study that assessed the relationship between coronary angiography and myocardial flow reserve, 29.1% of patients had a visual-functional mismatch, with 79.0% reporting an insignificant stenosis on coronary angiography but was functionally significant.[42] Therefore, additional functional or anatomic assessment should be considered when determining the need to revascularize the LMCA.

Physiologic assessment

Fractional flow reserve (FFR) is a physiologic test that can be used to determine the hemodynamic significance of a coronary artery stenosis. An FFR value of greater than 0.75 to 0.80 is generally accepted as a meaningful cutoff to determine a hemodynamically significant LMCA stenosis, based on the results of several studies that showed a high survival rate and a low cardiac event rate in LMCA patients treated with medical treatment who had an FFR greater than 0.75 to 0.80.[42–44] However, one should use clinical judgment in the interpretation of FFR. The value of FFR may increase if there is a lesion in the left anterior descending and/or left circumflex, which is the distal part of the LMCA. Therefore, one must correct for the disease location being in the distal part first and, then, reassess the functional significance.[45,46] FFR is also affected by elevated central venous pressure, inadequate response to

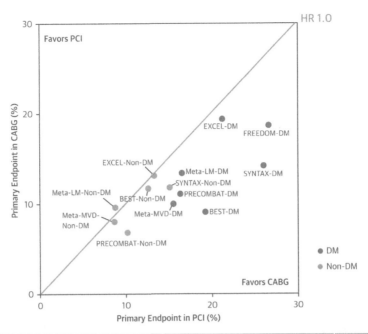

Fig. 1. Hazard ratio for the PCI compared with CABG for LMCA disease according to diabetic status.[34] BEST, comparison of coronary artery bypass surgery and everolimus-eluting stent implantation in the treatment of patients with multivessel coronary artery disease; DM, diabetes mellitus; FREEDOM, The Future Revascularization Evaluation in Patients with Diabetes Mellitus: Optimal Management of Multivessel Disease; IPD, individual patient-level data; LM, left main; NA, not available; TVR, target vessel revascularization.

Trial	Primary Endpoint	Hazard Ratio		p-Interaction
		DM	Non-DM	
Multivessel CAD				
SYNTAX (N = 1,800)	Composite of death, MI, stroke, or repeat revascularization	1.83 (1.22–2.73)	1.28 (0.97–1.69)	0.12
FREEDOM (N = 1,900)	Composite of death, MI, or stroke	<2 yr: 1.11 (0.85-1.45) >2 yr: 2.06 (1.41-3.02)	NA	NA
BEST (N = 880)	Composite of death, MI, or TVR	2.24 (1.25–4.00)	1.07 (0.65–1.76)	0.06
Left Main CAD				
PRECOMBAT (N = 600)	Composite of death, MI, stroke, or TVR	1.43 (0.65–3.16)	1.51 (0.76–2.99)	0.92
EXCEL (N = 1,905)	Composite of death, MI, or stroke	1.04 (0.70–1.55)	0.97 (0.72–1.30)	0.77
NOBLE (N = 1,184)	Composite of death, MI, stroke or repeat revascularization	15% DM, NA	NA	NA
IPD Meta-Analysis (11 RCT) (N = 11,518)				
Multivessel disease (N = 7,040)	All-cause death	1.48 (1.19–1.84)	1.08 (0.86–1.36)	0.045
Left main disease (N = 4,478)	All-cause death	1.34 (0.93–1.91)	0.94 (0.72–1.23)	0.13

adenosine, especially if the patient had recent ingestion of caffeine, and drift, which requires repeating FFR measurement after recalibration. The instantaneous wave-free ratio (iFR), a resting index of functional coronary stenosis, obviates the need for adenosine. Several studies support deferring revascularization if the iFR is greater than 0.89 except in LMCA disease.[47,48] However, without robust RCTs, the practical application of iFR in LMCA disease may be limited.

Intravascular ultrasound

Intravascular ultrasound (IVUS) is a useful device to assess the vessel diameter, minimum lumen area, lesion morphology, plaque burden, and plaque distribution. Previously, the MLA cutoff value for an abnormal FFR value in LMCA disease was 5.9 mm^2.[49] A multicenter study validated the MLA cutoff value less than 5.9 mm^2 based on Murray's law for proceeding with or deferring revascularization in intermediate LMCA disease.[50] In Korean patients with intermediate isolated ostial and/or shaft LMCA stenosis, an IVUS-derived MLA less than 4.5 mm^2 was identified as the cutoff value (77% sensitivity, 82% specificity, 84% positive predictive value, 75% negative predictive value, area under the curve: 0.83, 95% CI: 0.76–0.96; $P < .001$).[51] Variations in cutoff values can be due to differences in race, age, or coronary anatomy. Currently, an MLA greater than 6 mm^2 is considered a cutoff value for deferring revascularization for LMCA disease. IVUS is also used for stent optimization. Retrospective studies showed that IVUS-guided PCI for LMCA disease reduced mortality and in-stent restenosis.[52,53] Ongoing RCTs are being conducted to confirm the prognostic impact of IVUS-guided PCI in patients with LMCA disease.

PCI Technique

PCI strategy and techniques

PCI of the LMCA can be technically challenging as it commonly involves the distal bifurcation and is potentially riskier because of the large territory of myocardium that it subtends. Intravascular imaging and physiologic assessment with FFR should be routinely performed by a skilled interventionalist who has extensive experience in LMCA PCI, and emergent mechanical circulatory support should be available on standby in case the patient experiences hemodynamic collapse.[54] The treatment of an LMCA lesion located at the ostium or midshaft is relatively simple and associated with a lower MACE rate compared with a lesion located at the distal bifurcation.[55,56] However, the majority of LMCA disease involves the distal bifurcation. The presence or absence of a significant ostial left circumflex artery disease stenosis, which commonly supplies more than 10% of myocardial mass, plays a significant role in the selection of the stent technique.[57]

Two RCTs provided discordant results regarding whether a provisional stent approach or a 2-stent approach was the preferred technique for the treatment of distal bifurcation disease. In the Double Kissing Crush versus Provisional Stenting for Left Mian Distal Bifurcation Lesions (DKCRUSH-V) trial, a double-kissing (DK) crush 2-stent strategy resulted in a lower rate of target lesion failure (10.7% vs 5.0%; HR 0.42; 95% CI, 0.21–0.85; $P = .02$), target vessel MI (2.9% vs 0.4%; $P = .03$), and stent thrombosis (3.3% vs 0.4%; $P = .02$) at 12-month follow-up compared with a provisional strategy. The superior outcomes of the DK crush strategy were maintained at a 3-year follow-up.[58,59] In contrast, the European Bifurcation Club Left Main Study (EBC-MAIN) trial showed no significant difference in MACE, which was the composite of death, MI, and target lesion revascularization between the provisional one-stent group and the 2-stent group (14.7% vs 17.7%; HR 0.8; 95% CI, 0.5–1.3; $P = .34$). However, MACE was numerically lower with the provisional approach compared with a planned 2-stent approach[60] (Table 3).

The current consensus is that a single-stent crossover and provisional side-branch intervention is the preferred strategy for select cases with distal bifurcation disease that does not involve significant disease in the ostium of the left circumflex artery that is ≥ 2.5 mm in diameter.[61] Controversy surrounds the decision to treat asymptomatic patients with angiographic stenosis of the left circumflex artery after stenting the LMCA artery. Physiologic assessment of a jailed side branch with FFR can determine if it is hemodynamically significant and requires further revascularization to optimize the final angiographic result.[62,63]

In addition to the DK crush technique, other 2-stent techniques include the classic crush technique, culotte technique, and the T and protrusion technique. No RCT or guideline has clearly identified the preferred 2-stent technique for distal bifurcation disease. Therefore, the 2-stent technique can be selected at the discretion of the operator based on the bifurcation anatomy and the operator's experience. A network meta-analysis that compared 5 different bifurcation PCI techniques showed that the DK-crush technique was associated with a lower MACE rate, driven by a lower rate of repeat revascularization.[64] One limitation of the DK-crush technique is that it is technically challenging and requires an experienced operator.

Stent optimization

After stent implantation, intravascular imaging with IVUS or optical coherence tomography (OCT) can be used to optimize the final PCI results. IVUS may be the preferred intravascular imaging modality because OCT is not ideal in assessing the ostium of the LMCA. IVUS can identify stent

Table 3 Randomized controlled trials of stent technique for LMCA bifurcation disease	DK-CRUSH V Trial[58,59]	EBC-MAIN Trial[60]
Study design	Provisional strategy vs DK-Crush	Provisional strategy vs up-front 2-stent strategy
Recruitment period	2011–2016	2016–2019
N (provisional/2-stent)	242/240	230/237
Mean age (y)	64.5	71.1
Diabetes (%)	27.2	27.4
SYNTAX score, mean	30.6	22.9
Distal bifurcation angle (°)	78	81.3
Length of side branch lesion (mm)	16.4	6.9
Complex bifurcation (%)	31.5	Not classified
Operator experience	≥300 PCIs/y for 5 y, ≥20 left main PCIs/y	≥ 150 PCIs/y
Use of IVUS guidance (%)	Not mandated, 41.7	Not mandated, 32.5
Upfront 2-stent strategy	DK-crush	Culotte (53%), T/TAP (33%), DK-Crush (5%)
Conversion rate to 2-stent in provisional strategy (%)	47	22
Primary end point	TLF (composite of cardiac death, target vessel MI, or clinically driven TLR) at 1-y follow-up	Composite of all-cause death, MI, TLR at 1 y
Key findings	DK-Crush strategy lower rate of TLF at 1 and 3 y	No significant difference between the 2 strategies

Abbreviations: IVUS, intravascular ultrasound; TLF, target lesion failure; TLR, target lesion revascularization.

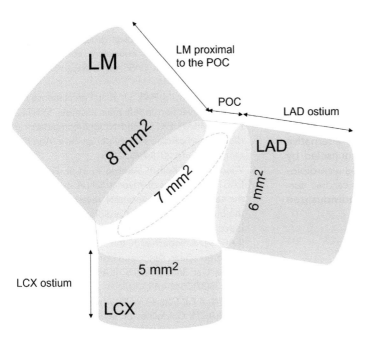

Fig. 2. IVUS-guided minimal stent area cutoff value for prevent in-stent restenosis (so-called 5-6-7-8 rule of criteria). LAD, left anterior descending artery; LCX, left circumflex artery, LM, left main.

underexpansion, malapposition, and edge dissection, resulting in improved clinical outcomes by reducing very late stent thrombosis and long-term mortality.[52] In the IVUS-TRONCO-ICP study, the incidence of cardiac death, MI, and target lesion revascularization, as well as stent thrombosis at 3 years was lower in the IVUS-guided group compared with the angiography-guided group.[53] To achieve optimal stent expansion to reduce the risk of in-stent restenosis, the minimal stent area should be at least 5.0 mm^2 for the left circumflex artery ostium, 6.3 mm^2 for the left anterior descending artery ostium, 7.2 mm^2 for the polygon of confluence, and 8.2 mm^2 for the proximal LMCA above the polygon of confluence ("5-6-7-8 rule")[65] (Fig. 2).

Hemodynamic support

During PCI for LMCA disease, balloon occlusion can induce global ischemia of the myocardium, resulting in life-threatening hemodynamic collapse. Fortunately, this is a rare occurrence in patients with normal LVEF, and prophylactic use of a mechanical circulatory support device is not indicated for most cases. However, mechanical circulatory support should be considered in patients with severe left ventricular dysfunction, critical right CAD, complex LMCA anatomy requiring atherectomy or a 2-stent technique, or hemodynamic instability.

SUMMARY

Over the past decade, advancements in PCI technology, intravascular imaging, which should be used in all cases, and routine use of physiologic assessment have led to improved PCI outcomes being on par with CABG in patients with LMCA disease and low or intermediate anatomic complexity. This has led to more widespread adoption of LMCA PCI in select patients. Results from landmark RCTs will likely lead to the revision of the guidelines on LMCA disease, which will recognize PCI as a reasonable alternative to CABG. The patient should be counseled by a Heart Team approach that includes a cardiologist working collaboratively with a cardiac surgeon to formulate an individualized revascularization strategy.

CLINICS CARE POINTS

- In the treatment of left main coronary artery disease, various factors, such as coronary artery complexity and possibility of complete revascularization, perioperative risk, and ejection fraction, should be considered.

- A multidisciplinary Heart Team approach with an informed decision should be recommended in intermediate left main coronary artery disease.

- In the left main coronary artery evaluation, active application of intravascular imaging and physiologic assessment should be considered.

REFERENCE

1. Lee PH, Ahn JM, Chang M, et al. Left main coronary artery disease: secular trends in patient characteristics, treatments, and outcomes. J Am Coll Cardiol 2016;68(11):1233–46.
2. Fihn SD, Blankenship JC, Alexander KP, et al. 2014 ACC/AHA/AATS/PCNA/SCAI/STS focused update of the guideline for the diagnosis and management of patients with stable ischemic heart disease: a report of the American College of Cardiology/American Heart Association Task Force on Practice Guidelines, and the American Association for Thoracic Surgery, Preventive Cardiovascular Nurses Association, Society for Cardiovascular Angiography and Interventions, and Society of Thoracic Surgeons. Circulation 2014;130(19):1749–67.
3. Takaro T, Hultgren HN, Lipton MJ, et al. The VA cooperative randomized study of surgery for coronary arterial occlusive disease II. Subgroup with significant left main lesions. Circulation 1976;54(6 Suppl):Iii107–17.
4. Caracciolo EA, Davis KB, Sopko G, et al. Comparison of surgical and medical group survival in patients with left main equivalent coronary artery disease. Long-term CASS experience. Circulation 1995;91(9):2335–44.
5. Park DW, Ahn JM, Park SJ, et al. Percutaneous coronary intervention in left main disease: SYNTAX, PRECOMBAT, EXCEL and NOBLE-combined cardiology and cardiac surgery perspective. Ann Cardiothorac Surg 2018;7(4):521–6.
6. Windecker S, Kolh P, Alfonso F, et al. 2014 ESC/EACTS Guidelines on myocardial revascularization: the task force on myocardial revascularization of the European Society of Cardiology (ESC) and the European Association for Cardio-Thoracic Surgery (EACTS)Developed with the special contribution of the European Association of Percutaneous Cardiovascular Interventions (EAPCI). Eur Heart J 2014;35(37):2541–619.
7. Neumann FJ, Sousa-Uva M, Ahlsson A, et al. 2018 ESC/EACTS Guidelines on myocardial revascularization. Eur Heart J 2019;40(2):87–165.

8. Lawton JS, Tamis-Holland JE, Bangalore S, et al. 2021 ACC/AHA/SCAI guideline for coronary artery revascularization: a report of the American College of Cardiology/American Heart Association Joint Committee on Clinical Practice Guidelines. J Am Coll Cardiol 2021;79(2):e21–129.

9. Buszman PE, Kiesz SR, Bochenek A, et al. Acute and late outcomes of unprotected left main stenting in comparison with surgical revascularization. J Am Coll Cardiol 2008;51(5):538–45.

10. Morice MC, Serruys PW, Kappetein AP, et al. Outcomes in patients with de novo left main disease treated with either percutaneous coronary intervention using paclitaxel-eluting stents or coronary artery bypass graft treatment in the Synergy Between Percutaneous Coronary Intervention with TAXUS and Cardiac Surgery (SYNTAX) trial. Circulation 2010;121(24):2645–53.

11. Park SJ, Kim YH, Park DW, et al. Randomized trial of stents versus bypass surgery for left main coronary artery disease. N Engl J Med 2011;364(18):1718–27.

12. Boudriot E, Thiele H, Walther T, et al. Randomized comparison of percutaneous coronary intervention with sirolimus-eluting stents versus coronary artery bypass grafting in unprotected left main stem stenosis. J Am Coll Cardiol 2011;57(5):538–45.

13. Buszman PE, Buszman PP, Banasiewicz-Szkróbka I, et al. Left main stenting in comparison with surgical revascularization: 10-year outcomes of the (left main coronary artery stenting) LE MANS trial. JACC Cardiovasc Interv 2016;9(4):318–27.

14. Park DW, Ahn JM, Park H, et al. Ten-year outcomes after drug-eluting stents versus coronary artery bypass grafting for left main coronary disease: extended follow-up of the PRECOMBAT trial. Circulation 2020;141(18):1437–46.

15. Morice MC, Serruys PW, Kappetein AP, et al. Five-year outcomes in patients with left main disease treated with either percutaneous coronary intervention or coronary artery bypass grafting in the synergy between percutaneous coronary intervention with taxus and cardiac surgery trial. Circulation 2014;129(23):2388–94.

16. Stone GW, Sabik JF, Serruys PW, et al. Everolimus-eluting stents or bypass surgery for left main coronary artery disease. N Engl J Med 2016;375(23):2223–35.

17. Stone GW, Kappetein AP, Sabik JF, et al. Five-year outcomes after PCI or CABG for left main coronary disease. N Engl J Med 2019;381(19):1820–30.

18. Mäkikallio T, Holm NR, Lindsay M, et al. Percutaneous coronary angioplasty versus coronary artery bypass grafting in treatment of unprotected left main stenosis (NOBLE): a prospective, randomised, open-label, non-inferiority trial. Lancet 2016;388(10061):2743–52.

19. Holm NR, Mäkikallio T, Lindsay MM, et al. Percutaneous coronary angioplasty versus coronary artery bypass grafting in the treatment of unprotected left main stenosis: updated 5-year outcomes from the randomised, non-inferiority NOBLE trial. Lancet 2020;395(10219):191–9.

20. Head SJ, Milojevic M, Daemen J, et al. Mortality after coronary artery bypass grafting versus percutaneous coronary intervention with stenting for coronary artery disease: a pooled analysis of individual patient data. Lancet 2018;391(10124):939–48.

21. Athappan G, Patvardhan E, Tuzcu ME, et al. Left main coronary artery stenosis: a meta-analysis of drug-eluting stents versus coronary artery bypass grafting. JACC Cardiovasc Interv 2013;6(12):1219–30.

22. Giacoppo D, Colleran R, Cassese S, et al. Percutaneous coronary intervention vs coronary artery bypass grafting in patients with left main coronary artery stenosis: a systematic review and meta-analysis. JAMA Cardiol 2017;2(10):1079–88.

23. Upadhaya S, Baniya R, Madala S, et al. Drug-eluting stent placement versus coronary artery bypass surgery for unprotected left main coronary artery disease: a meta-analysis of randomized controlled trials. J Card Surg 2017;32(2):70–9.

24. Ahmad Y, Howard JP, Arnold AD, et al. Mortality after drug-eluting stents vs. coronary artery bypass grafting for left main coronary artery disease: a meta-analysis of randomized controlled trials. Eur Heart J 2020;41(34):3228–35.

25. Kuno T, Ueyama H, Rao SV, et al. Percutaneous coronary intervention or coronary artery bypass graft surgery for left main coronary artery disease: A meta-analysis of randomized trials. Am Heart J 2020;227:9–10.

26. Sianos G, Morel MA, Kappetein AP, et al. The SYNTAX Score: an angiographic tool grading the complexity of coronary artery disease. EuroIntervention 2005;1(2):219–27.

27. Yoon YH, Ahn JM, Kang DY, et al. Impact of SYNTAX Score on 10-Year Outcomes After Revascularization for Left Main Coronary Artery Disease. JACC Cardiovasc Interv 2020;13(3):361–71.

28. Farooq V, Serruys PW, Garcia-Garcia HM, et al. The negative impact of incomplete angiographic revascularization on clinical outcomes and its association with total occlusions: the SYNTAX (Synergy Between Percutaneous Coronary Intervention with Taxus and Cardiac Surgery) trial. J Am Coll Cardiol 2013;61(3):282–94.

29. Lee J, Ahn JM, Kim JH, et al. Prognostic effect of the SYNTAX score on 10-year outcomes after left main coronary artery revascularization in a randomized population: insights from the extended PRECOMBAT trial. J Am Heart Assoc 2021;10(14):e020359.

30. Nashef SA, Roques F, Sharples LD, et al. Euro-SCORE II. Eur J Cardiothorac Surg 2012;41(4):734–44 [discussion: 744-735].

31. Farooq V, van Klaveren D, Steyerberg EW, et al. Anatomical and clinical characteristics to guide decision making between coronary artery bypass surgery and percutaneous coronary intervention for individual patients: development and validation of SYNTAX score II. Lancet 2013;381(9867):639–50.

32. Takahashi K, Serruys PW, Fuster V, et al. Redevelopment and validation of the SYNTAX score II to individualise decision making between percutaneous and surgical revascularisation in patients with complex coronary artery disease: secondary analysis of the multicentre randomised controlled SYNTAXES trial with external cohort validation. Lancet 2020;396(10260):1399–412.

33. Farkouh ME, Domanski M, Sleeper LA, et al. Strategies for multivessel revascularization in patients with diabetes. N Engl J Med 2012;367(25):2375–84.

34. Park SJ, Park DW. Diabetes in myocardial revascularization for left main coronary artery disease: predictor or decision maker? J Am Coll Cardiol 2019;73(13):1629–32.

35. Milojevic M, Serruys PW, Sabik JF 3rd, et al. Bypass surgery or stenting for left main coronary artery disease in patients with diabetes. J Am Coll Cardiol 2019;73(13):1616–28.

36. Lee K, Ahn JM, Yoon YH, et al. Long-Term (10-Year) outcomes of stenting or bypass surgery for left main coronary artery disease in patients with and without diabetes mellitus. J Am Heart Assoc 2020;9(8):e015372.

37. Takaro T, Peduzzi P, Detre KM, et al. Survival in subgroups of patients with left main coronary artery disease. Veterans administration cooperative study of surgery for coronary arterial occlusive disease. Circulation 1982;66(1):14–22.

38. Wolff G, Dimitroulis D, Andreotti F, et al. Survival benefits of invasive versus conservative strategies in heart failure in patients with reduced ejection fraction and coronary artery disease: a meta-analysis. Circ Heart Fail 2017;10(1):e003255.

39. Park S, Ahn JM, Kim TO, et al. Revascularization in Patients with left main coronary artery disease and left ventricular dysfunction. J Am Coll Cardiol 2020;76(12):1395–406.

40. Mesana T, Rodger N, Sherrard H. Heart teams: a new paradigm in health care. Can J Cardiol 2018;34(7):815–8.

41. Lindstaedt M, Spiecker M, Perings C, et al. How good are experienced interventional cardiologists at predicting the functional significance of intermediate or equivocal left main coronary artery stenoses? Int J Cardiol 2007;120(2):254–61.

42. Hamilos M, Muller O, Cuisset T, et al. Long-term clinical outcome after fractional flow reserve-guided treatment in patients with angiographically equivocal left main coronary artery stenosis. Circulation 2009;120(15):1505–12.

43. Zahn R, Hamm CW, Schneider S, et al. Predictors of death or myocardial infarction during follow-up after coronary stenting with the sirolimus-eluting stent. Results from the prospective multicenter German Cypher Stent Registry. Am Heart J 2006;152(6):1146–52.

44. Courtis J, Rodés-Cabau J, Larose E, et al. Usefulness of coronary fractional flow reserve measurements in guiding clinical decisions in intermediate or equivocal left main coronary stenoses. Am J Cardiol 2009;103(7):943–9.

45. Park SJ, Ahn JM, Kang SJ. Unprotected left main percutaneous coronary intervention: integrated use of fractional flow reserve and intravascular ultrasound. J Am Heart Assoc 2012;1(6):e004556.

46. Kim HL, Koo BK, Nam CW, et al. Clinical and physiological outcomes of fractional flow reserve-guided percutaneous coronary intervention in patients with serial stenoses within one coronary artery. JACC Cardiovasc Interv 2012;5(10):1013–8.

47. Götberg M, Christiansen EH, Gudmundsdottir IJ, et al. Instantaneous Wave-free Ratio versus Fractional Flow Reserve to Guide PCI. N Engl J Med 2017;376(19):1813–23.

48. Davies JE, Sen S, Dehbi HM, et al. Use of the Instantaneous Wave-free Ratio or Fractional Flow Reserve in PCI. N Engl J Med 2017;376(19):1824–34.

49. Jasti V, Ivan E, Yalamanchili V, et al. Correlations between fractional flow reserve and intravascular ultrasound in patients with an ambiguous left main coronary artery stenosis. Circulation 2004;110(18):2831–6.

50. de la Torre Hernandez JM, Hernández Hernandez F, Alfonso F, et al. Prospective application of pre-defined intravascular ultrasound criteria for assessment of intermediate left main coronary artery lesions results from the multicenter LITRO study. J Am Coll Cardiol 2011;58(4):351–8.

51. Park SJ, Ahn JM, Kang SJ, et al. Intravascular ultrasound-derived minimal lumen area criteria for functionally significant left main coronary artery stenosis. JACC Cardiovasc Interv 2014;7(8):868–74.

52. Park SJ, Kim YH, Park DW, et al. Impact of intravascular ultrasound guidance on long-term mortality in stenting for unprotected left main coronary artery stenosis. Circ Cardiovasc Interv 2009;2(3):167–77.

53. de la Torre Hernandez JM, Baz Alonso JA, Gómez Hospital JA, et al. Clinical impact of intravascular ultrasound guidance in drug-eluting stent implantation for unprotected left main coronary disease: pooled analysis at the patient-level of 4 registries. JACC Cardiovasc Interv 2014;7(3):244–54.

54. Xu B, Redfors B, Yang Y, et al. Impact of Operator Experience and Volume on Outcomes After Left

Main Coronary Artery Percutaneous Coronary Intervention. JACC Cardiovasc Interv 2016;9(20):2086–93.

55. Chieffo A, Park SJ, Valgimigli M, et al. Favorable long-term outcome after drug-eluting stent implantation in nonbifurcation lesions that involve unprotected left main coronary artery: a multicenter registry. Circulation 2007;116(2):158–62.

56. Naganuma T, Chieffo A, Meliga E, et al. Long-term clinical outcomes after percutaneous coronary intervention for ostial/mid-shaft lesions versus distal bifurcation lesions in unprotected left main coronary artery: the DELTA Registry (drug-eluting stent for left main coronary artery disease): a multicenter registry evaluating percutaneous coronary intervention versus coronary artery bypass grafting for left main treatment. JACC Cardiovasc Interv 2013;6(12):1242–9.

57. Kim HY, Doh JH, Lim HS, et al. Identification of coronary artery side branch supplying myocardial mass that may benefit from revascularization. JACC Cardiovasc Interv 2017;10(6):571–81.

58. Chen SL, Zhang JJ, Han Y, et al. Double kissing crush versus provisional stenting for left main distal bifurcation lesions: DKCRUSH-V randomized trial. J Am Coll Cardiol 2017;70(21):2605–17.

59. Chen X, Li X, Zhang JJ, et al. 3-Year Outcomes of the DKCRUSH-V trial comparing dk crush with provisional stenting for left main bifurcation lesions. JACC Cardiovasc Interv 2019;12(19):1927–37.

60. Hildick-Smith D, Egred M, Banning A, et al. The European bifurcation club Left Main Coronary Stent study: a randomized comparison of stepwise provisional vs. systematic dual stenting strategies (EBC MAIN). Eur Heart J 2021;42(37):3829–39.

61. Burzotta F, Lassen JF, Lefèvre T, et al. Percutaneous coronary intervention for bifurcation coronary lesions: the 15(th) consensus document from the European Bifurcation Club. EuroIntervention 2021;16(16):1307–17.

62. Koo BK, Kang HJ, Youn TJ, et al. Physiologic assessment of jailed side branch lesions using fractional flow reserve. J Am Coll Cardiol 2005;46(4):633–7.

63. Lee CH, Choi SW, Hwang J, et al. 5-Year outcomes according to FFR of left circumflex coronary artery after left main crossover stenting. JACC Cardiovasc Interv 2019;12(9):847–55.

64. Di Gioia G, Sonck J, Ferenc M, et al. Clinical outcomes following coronary bifurcation pci techniques: a systematic review and network meta-analysis comprising 5,711 patients. JACC Cardiovasc Interv 2020;13(12):1432–44.

65. Kang SJ, Ahn JM, Song H, et al. Comprehensive intravascular ultrasound assessment of stent area and its impact on restenosis and adverse cardiac events in 403 patients with unprotected left main disease. Circ Cardiovasc Interv 2011;4(6):562–9.

Calcium Modification in Percutaneous Coronary Interventions

Richard A. Shlofmitz, MD[a],*,
Keyvan Karimi Galougahi, MD, PhD[a],
Allen Jeremias, MD, MSc[a,b], Evan Shlofmitz, DO[a],
Susan V. Thomas, MPH[a], Ziad A. Ali, MD, DPhil[a,b]

KEYWORDS

- Coronary calcification • Intravascular ultrasound • Optical coherence tomography
- Rotational atherectomy • Orbital atherectomy • Intravascular lithotripsy

KEY POINTS

- Severe lesion calcification increases the complexity of percutaneous coronary intervention (PCI) and is associated with suboptimal procedural and long-term outcomes.
- Intravascular imaging prior to intervention is key in the assessment of calcification type and severity.
- Guided by intravascular imaging, various calcium modification modalities can be used in an algorithmic approach to effectively modify calcium.
- Documentation of calcium fracture on intravascular imaging prior to stent implantation is important to ensure achieving optimal minimal stent area.
- Intravascular imaging assessment is essential in understanding the mechanism of in-stent restenosis in the presence of calcification and selection of appropriate calcium modification techniques.

INTRODUCTION

Calcification poses several challenges to the treatment of coronary stenoses by percutaneous coronary intervention (PCI) because the rigid calcific plaques are difficult to cross and dilate by interventional devices. There are several modalities available to treat calcified coronary arteries.[1] Prior to deciding which treatment is best or even needed, one needs to assess the target lesion and the vessel with intravascular imaging. Angiography alone is not adequate in assessing the morphologic characteristics of calcium in coronary lesions.[2]

Historically, calcium ablative procedures were used as bail out in situations where a balloon could not cross or dilate a lesion. This approach was effective in completing the procedures but did not necessarily result in optimal initial or long-term results.[3,4] By utilizing intravascular imaging in an algorithmic approach, one can plan logically if ablative techniques are necessary and if so, which is best suited for a specific target lesion.[1]

INTRAVASCULAR IMAGING GUIDANCE FOR CALCIUM MODIFICATION

Intravascular imaging is key in determining the morphology of the target coronary lesion (**Fig. 1**). On optical coherence tomography (OCT), 3 types of atherosclerotic plaques can be identified: fibrous plaques, lipid-rich plaques, and calcified plaques (see **Fig. 1**). Lesion

[a] Staint Francis Hospital & Heart Center, 100 Port Washington Boulevard, Roslyn, NY 11576, USA;
[b] Cardiovascular Research Foundation, 1700 Broadway, New York, NY 10019, USA
* Corresponding author.
E-mail address: Richard.Shlofmitz@CHSLI.org

Intervent Cardiol Clin 11 (2022) 373–381
https://doi.org/10.1016/j.iccl.2022.06.001

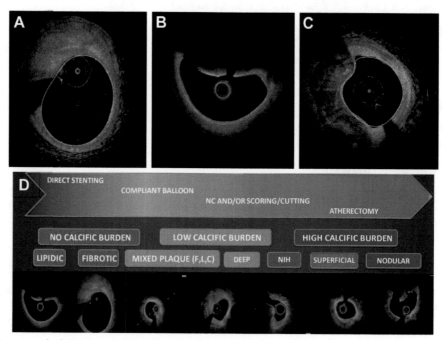

Fig. 1. *Assessment of plaque morphology by optical coherence tomography. (A) Fibrotic plaque, (B), lipid-rich pla-que, (C) calcified plaque. (D). Plaque modification strategies tailored to specific plaque types on optical coherence tomography. C, calcific; F, fibrotic; L, lipidic; NC, non-compliant; NIH, neointimal hyperplasia.*

preparation strategies can then be targeted to the specific types of morphologies and calcification burden, ranging from direct stenting to semi-compliant balloon dilatation, noncompliant or scoring/cutting balloon dilatation or atherectomy (see Fig. 1).

In intravascular imaging, there are 3 types of calcified coronary plaques (see Fig. 1): 1 - deep calcium, where calcium is located deep in the arterial wall and covered by superficial fibrosis adjacent to the lumen. The deep calcification usually can be treated with conventional or specialty balloons; 2 - nodular calcium, which protrudes into the lumen. Protruding calcified nodules with a disrupted fibrous cap can be associated with platelet aggregation and act similar to the disrupted thin cap fibroatheroma as a cause for acute coronary syndromes.[5] They are not usually successfully treated with the balloon technology and require ablative techniques; 3 - superficial calcium, this occurs when calcium has no or minimal fibrotic layer near the lumen. Successful treatment of superficial calcium depends on the thickness, length, and arc of calcium that represent the three-dimensional volume of the calcific deposit.[6]

If the calcium thickness is greater than 0.5 mm and the arc is greater than 50% of vessel circumference (180°) with the length greater than 5 mm, conventional balloons are not usually effective in adequately modifying calcium and resulting in optimal minimal stent area, and ablative techniques are recommended.[6,7] An OCT-based calcium score reflecting these volumetric measurements of calcium has been developed and validated with 2 points for maximum calcium angle >180°, 1 point for maximum calcium thickness >0.5 mm, and 1 point for calcium length >5 mm, for a total calcium score of 0–4 points (see Fig. 1).[7] Stent expansion was 99% (interquartile range [IQR]: 93–108) in lesions with score 0, 85% [78–93] with score 1, 86% [77–100] with score 2, 80% [73–85] with score 3, and 78% [70–86] with score 4; p < 0.01.[7] Therefore, OCT-based calcium score of ≥3 may indicate the need for calcium modification to induce calcium fracture, which is associated with enhanced stent expansion.[6] Fig. 2 presents an example where a combination of the calcium measurement indices was present on OCT of a severely calcified lesion, mandating calcium modification with an ablative technique. These morphologic characteristics are integrated into an algorithmic approach to select the best technique that is tailored for a specific calcified plaque morphology. Fig. 3 presents a flow chart on how to use intravascular imaging, in particular OCT, to guide calcium modification, with the aim of inducing calcium fracture that facilitates optimal stent expansion.

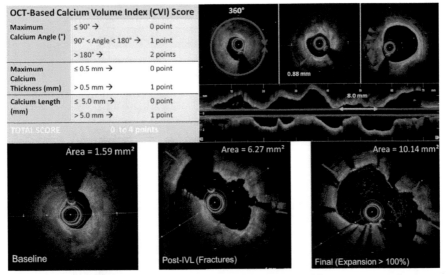

Fig. 2. *Assessment of a severely calcified lesion and impact of calcium modification on optical coherence tomography (OCT). A circumference of 360, thickness of 0.88 mm, and a calcium length of 8.0 mm add to a score of 4, suggesting that calcium modification is needed for optimal stenting results. Intravascular lithotripsy (IVL) is performed, leading to multiple deep fractures (arrows), leading to excellent stent expansion.*

IN-STENT RESTENOSIS DUE TO CALCIFICATION

In addition to de novo coronary lesions, in-stent restenosis is also frequently due to calcification. Stent under expansion may be secondary to inadequate calcium modification without inducing calcium fracture during the index procedure leading to suboptimal minimal stent area.[8] Neo-intimal hyperplasia with calcification is also observed after the implantation of drug-eluting stents, especially after 20 months since implantation.[9,10] Both of these situations can only be assessed with intravascular imaging.

Fig. 4 presents a flow chart based on intravascular imaging to guide the assessment and targeted treatment of in-stent restenosis. A step-by-step approach is provided that takes into account the presence or absence of calcium behind the struts or in the neointimal tissue on OCT, and possibility for balloon crossing and dilatation. Combined, these characteristics plus the morphology of calcium on OCT guide the selection of appropriate calcium modification modalities to treat in-stent restenosis.

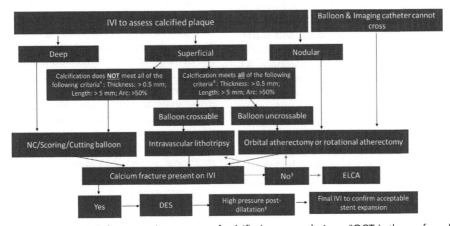

Fig. 3. *Algorithmic approach for optimal treatment of calcified coronary lesions. [a]OCT is the preferred imaging modality for the comprehensive assessment of calcified lesions given its unique ability to assess calcium thickness. DES, drug-eluting stent; ELCA, excimer laser coronary atherectomy; IVI, intravascular imaging; NC, noncompliant; OCT, optical coherence tomography. ‡, >12 atm.*

OCT APPROACH TO RESTENOSIS

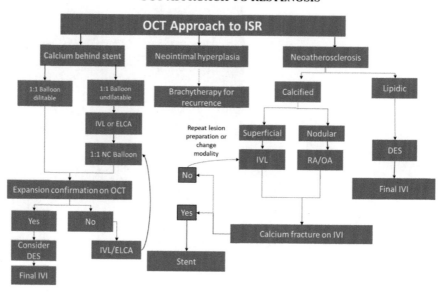

Fig. 4. *Treatment of in-stent restenosis with optical coherence tomography guidance.* DES, drug-eluting stent; ELCA, excimer laser coronary atherectomy; ISR, in-stent restenosis; IVI, intravascular imaging; IVL, intravascular lithotripsy; NC, noncompliant; OA, orbital atherectomy; OCT, optical coherence tomography; RA, rotational atherectomy.

CALCIUM MODIFICATION MODALITIES

Table 1 lists the specific features and comparison of 4 available calcium modification modalities and their relative advantages and disadvantages.

Intravascular Lithotripsy

Intravascular lithotripsy (IVL) (Shockwave Medical, Santa Clara, CA) impacts calcium with expanding and collapsing vapor bubbles that create a short burst of acoustic pressure waves.[11] These pressure waves travel through the vessel tissue with an effective pressure of 50 atm. There is a localized field effect in the vessel wall, which creates both deep and superficial calcium fracture.[11] This technique requires minimal setup by the staff. The coronary IVL balloon catheter is 12 mm in length with sizes ranging from 2.5 to 4.00 mm. There are 80 pulses available per catheter. IVL is advanced over a "workhorse wire." Generally, if the lesion can be crossed with a "specialty balloon," IVL balloon will also cross the calcified target lesion. IVL works well using a 1:1 ratio of balloon to vessel size and when there is > 180° of calcium present.

IVL is ideal for bifurcation lesions including in left main coronary disease as the operator can wire and protect both major branches during lesion preparation. There is no downstream debris released; therefore, hemodynamics and rhythm remain stable during shock wave delivery.[12] Based on intravascular imaging assessment, the 80 pulses available per catheter should be applied to the coronary segments requiring the most calcium modification. IVL is an easy, safe and effective technology with the high cost being a potential issue at present.

ORBITAL ATHERECTOMY

Orbital Atherectomy (OA) (Cardiovascular Systems, Inc., St. Paul, Minnesota) provides safe and effective treatment to change the compliance of severely calcified coronary lesions.[13,14] OA uses a differential sanding mechanism to reduce calcified plaque volume while minimizing the damage to the noncalcified tissue.[15] The OA system is equipped with a 1.25 mm eccentrically mounted diamond-coated crown connected to a drive shaft and to a controller powered by a pneumatic console that allows for the bidirectional modification of calcium at 80,000 or 120,000 rpm. By increasing its elliptical orbit as rotational speed increases, OA allows for the ablation of calcium using the same device (1.25-mm crown) in vessels up to 3.5 mm in diameter. The elliptical orbit allows blood and microdebris to flow past the crown, continually dispersing the particulate, cooling the crown, and reducing the risk of thermal injury and decreasing ischemia and distal embolization.

Table 1
Technical features and clinical indication of calcium modification modalities

	Rotational Atherectomy	Coronary Orbital Atherectomy	Intravascular Lithotripsy (IVL)	Excimer Laser Coronary Atherectomy (ELCA)
Mechanism of Action	Rotational Diamond-tipped burr spins concentrically on the wire Atheroablation via sanding/abrasion	Orbital Eccentrically mounted diamond-coated crown uses centrifugal force to orbit, allowing for continuous blood flow during the procedure Atheroablation via sanding/abrasion	Acoustic pressure waves	Laser Multifiber laser catheters transmit ultra-violet energy Photoablation (vaporization)
Clinical Indication	A sole therapy or adjunctive balloon angioplasty is indicated in patients with coronary artery disease who are acceptable candidates for coronary artery bypass graft surgery.	To facilitate stent delivery in patients with coronary artery disease who are acceptable candidates for PTCA or stenting due to de novo, severely calcified coronary artery lesions. OAS is approved by the US FDA for the treatment of de novo, severely calcified lesions in the coronary arteries.	Heavily calcified (>270°) de novo coronary lesions	A stand-alone modality or in conjunction with PTCA in patients who are acceptable candidates for coronary artery bypass graft surgery. • Moderately calcified lesions • In-stent restenosis of stainless steel stents • Saphenous vein grafts
Technical Features	Front-cutting, mono-directional burr	Diamond coated crown, bidirectional treatment	Expanding and collapsing vapor bubble creates a short burst of acoustic pressure waves. Has an effective pressure of ~50 atm	Over the wire and rapid exchange catheters
	Multiple burr sizes (8) 1.25 to 2.5 mm	1.25 mm classic crown orbits to treats larger diameter	1:1 sizing: multiple balloon sizes ranging from 2.5 to 4.0 mm in 12 mm lengths	Available with concentric and eccentric tip designs
	0.009″/0.014″ tip RotaWire Guide Wires		0.014″ Guidewire	0.014″ Guidewire

(continued on next page)

Table 1
(continued)

	Rotational Atherectomy	Coronary Orbital Atherectomy	Intravascular Lithotripsy (IVL)	Excimer Laser Coronary Atherectomy (ELCA)
		0.012"/0.014" tip ViperWire Advance Coronary Guide Wire		
	Speed: ranging from 140krpm to 180krpm during treatment	Speeds: 80krpm, 120krpm	Therapeutic inflation of 4 atms to have contact with vessel – minimize barotrauma and nominal pressure of 6 atms; 80 pulses total at 1 pulse/sec for 8 cycles	Adjustable laser energy settings
Advantages	Easy staff setup Ideal for nodular calcium and balloon uncrossable lesions Sanding antegrade and retrograde – reduce burr entrapment and ostial lesion Glide assist to deliver distal to lesion, retrograde sanding, and device removal	Possible for single operator Dedicated guide wire is highly torquable High success rate in *de novo* complex calcific and balloon uncrossable lesion and ISR (neo-calcification and double-layer stent under expansion) Choice device for tortuous lesion segment Dynaglide use for distal delivery, device removal, and single operator use	Easy use and setup by physician and staff Ideal for bifurcation lesion; maintain wire position in both branches Ability to cross similar to specialty balloons Minimal hemodynamic changes	Easy use by physician Can be used on any workhorse wire Ideal for ISR underexpansion and uncrossable lesions Moderate debulking for neointimal hyperplasia
Disadvantages	Must be used with an experienced operator Less effective for deep calcium Increased risk of perforation in angulated and tortuous vessels Cannot be used with second wire in the side branch Must be used with ViperWire – equivalent to workhorse	Do not use with second wire in side branch	Fractures calcium but does not ablate With long calcified lesions, may need to use multiple IVL catheters Best if ≥ 270° of calcium	Cumbersome staff setup Risk of dissection with *de novo* lesions Increased effectiveness if used by a knowledgeable operator with off-label contrast flush use

OA has a fully operator-controlled electric console that facilitates rapid setup. The 6 Fr compatible ViperWire Advance with flex tip is a hydrophobic silicone-coated wire with nitinol core and a radiopaque distal spring tip, which is used exclusively to advance the OA crown. The ViperWire Advance is torquable and tracks well, with its flexibility reducing wire bias. OA at the glide assist mode uses a low rotational crown speed (5000 rpm) to facilitate crossing the ostial lesions, traversing long tortuous lesions, and for device removal.[16]

Once the wire is in the proper position and the advancer knob is locked at the 1-cm mark, the crown is advanced to approximately 5 mm proximal to the lesion. If the lesion is severely stenosed, it may be useful to place the nose cone of the device partially into the lesion to facilitate crossing. OA activation is by a simple push of a button on the sled. After relieving tension by unlocking and sliding the advancer knob to the 0-cm mark, slow and steady advancement at 1 mm/s traverse rate results in a larger luminal gain compared with advancement at 10 mm/s[17] Rapid advancement (>10 mm/s) may increase the risk of dissections and perforations.

The device works bidirectionally, and it is important to use the same slow movement when advancing the crown forward or backward. Adequate ablation is achieved when there is no resistance to crown movement and no change in pitch/sound is perceived resulting from crown contact with calcium in the wall of the artery. It is recommended that run time should not exceed 30 s. The low-speed mode (80,000 rpm) should be used for the initial pass. Most lesions treated with OA do not require the high-speed mode (120,000 rpm). The high-speed mode should be avoided in tortuous segments, severe angulations, and vessels smaller than 3.0 mm. The high-speed mode should only be used when there is insufficient ablation or compliance change after 2 or more runs at the low-speed mode.

ROTATIONAL ATHERECTOMY

The Rotablator system (Boston Scientific, Marlborough, Massachusetts) ablates calcified plaques using a diamond-encrusted elliptical burr, rotated at speeds of 140,000 to 190,000 rpm by a helical driveshaft that is advanced across the lesion over a guidewire.[18] The burr causes "differential cutting" and preferentially ablates the hard, inelastic, calcified plaque that does not stretch away from the RA burr compared with the healthy arterial tissue.[18]

RA was approved by the US Food and Drug Administration for use in 1993 and has the longest clinical application to-date of all the ablative techniques. RA use was previously limited by the difficult set up by staff as well as for the operator. The upgraded contemporary device, RotaPro (Boston Scientific, Marlborough, Massachusetts), has many improved features including a console that does not require a bulky gas tank, an improved wire, table side controls instead of a foot pedal, and the ability to dynaglide in and out of the catheter and vessel by a single operator.

Techniques for RA have changed over the years to improve procedural success, including using slower speeds (150,000 rpm), observation for deceleration, and careful selection of the burr size. RA with 1.25–2.5 mm burr is ideal for superficial calcified lesions that are long and in tortuous segments. RA is most operators' choice for balloon uncrossable lesions. RA can be very effective in in-stent restenosis both with neointimal calcification and in double-layers of stents. Bifurcation lesions have to be treated individually; therefore, side branch protection can be an issue.

EXCIMER LASER CORONARY ATHERECTOMY

Excimer laser coronary atherectomy (ELCA) using the CVX-300 cardiovascular laser Excimer system (Philips, Amsterdam, Netherlands) debulks and modifies the tissue with its photochemical, photothermal, and photokinetic properties without causing significant tissue injury.[19] ELCA is an important tool that allows for the completion of difficult and complicated cases. It is a useful tool for uncrossable or undilatable lesions. Application of laser in blood or contrast media is rarely performed in de novo lesions due to concerns regarding uncontrolled plaque modification, which can lead to dissection and perforation, and is limited to specific situations such as the treatment of under-expanded stents within severely calcified lesions.[20] Accumulating evidence supports the efficacy of this approach using ELCA in such cases of under-expanded stents.[21,22] In addition, ELCA is increasingly used for chronic total occlusion (CTO) PCI to facilitate the modification of the proximal CTO cap to allow penetration.[20,23]

Setup of the device by staff has been cumbersome but the new iteration of the device has significant advances, making utilization acceptable. Actual use of the device is easy for the operator using a workhorse wire and is similar to passing any balloon catheter. Coronary catheters are available in 4 diameters, 0.9 mm (6F-compatible), 1.4 mm and 1.7 mm (7F-compatible), and 2.0 mm (8F-compatible). For resistant calcified in-stent lesions, a progression of ELCA catheter sizes may be necessary to achieve acceptable results.

SUMMARY

Intravascular imaging is the only way to assess the type and severity of calcified coronary lesions and should be performed prior to PCI. Once the type and severity of calcium are established, a logical choice of equipment can be made to achieve optimal results. Regardless of which technique is chosen to modify calcium, one should always image prior to stent implantation to document calcium fracture and perform final imaging poststent to assess the stent expansion and exclude stent edge dissection. PCI on severely calcified lesions is one of the most challenging procedures in interventional cardiology and is associated with increased acute and chronic complications. Therefore, comprehensive assessment before and after PCI in heavily calcified lesions is critical to obtain optimal results.

CLINICS CARE POINTS

- Calcification inhibits adequate stent expansion.
- Stent expansion is an important predictor of future events-Intravascular imaging can guide optimal lesion preparation.

DISCLOSURE

R.A. Shlofmitz is a consultant for Shockwave Medical. E. Shlofmitz is a consultant for Abbott Vascular, ACIST Medical, Boston Scientific, Cardiovascular Systems, Inc., Janssen Pharmaceuticals, Medtronic, OpSens Medical, Philips, and Shockwave Medical.

REFERENCES

1. Karimi Galougahi K, Shlofmitz E, Jeremias A, et al. Therapeutic approach to calcified coronary lesions: disruptive technologies. current cardiology reports. Curr Cardiol Rep 2021;23(4):33.
2. Copeland-Halperin RS, Baber U, Aquino M, et al. Prevalence, correlates, and impact of coronary calcification on adverse events following PCI with newer-generation DES: Findings from a large multiethnic registry. Catheter Cardiovasc Interv 2018; 91(5):859–66.
3. Bourantas CV, Zhang YJ, Garg S, et al. Prognostic implications of coronary calcification in patients with obstructive coronary artery disease treated by percutaneous coronary intervention: a patient-level pooled analysis of 7 contemporary stent trials. Heart 2014;100(15):1158–64.
4. Huisman J, van der Heijden LC, Kok MM, et al. Impact of severe lesion calcification on clinical outcome of patients with stable angina, treated with newer generation permanent polymer-coated drug-eluting stents: a patient-level pooled analysis from TWENTE and DUTCH PEERS (TWENTE II). Am Heart J 2016;175:121–9.
5. Prati F, Gatto L, Fabbiocchi F, et al. Clinical outcomes of calcified nodules detected by optical coherence tomography: a sub-analysis of the CLIMA study. EuroIntervention 2020;16(5):380–6.
6. Ali ZA, Galougahi KK. Shining light on calcified lesions, plaque stabilisation and physiologic significance: new insights from intracoronary OCT. EuroIntervention 2018;13(18):e2105–8.
7. Fujino A, Mintz GS, Matsumura M, et al. A new optical coherence tomography-based calcium scoring system to predict stent underexpansion. EuroIntervention 2018;13(18):e2182–9.
8. Dong Y, Mintz G, Song L, et al. In-stent restenosis lesion morphology related to new stent underexpansion as evaluated by optical coherence tomography. J Am Coll Cardiol 2017;70(Supplement 18): B236.
9. Song L, Mintz GS, Yin D, et al. Characteristics of early versus late in-stent restenosis in second-generation drug-eluting stents: an optical coherence tomography study. EuroIntervention 2017; 13(3):294–302.
10. Kang SJ, Mintz GS, Akasaka T, et al. Optical coherence tomographic analysis of in-stent neoatherosclerosis after drug-eluting stent implantation. Circulation 2011;123(25):2954–63.
11. Karimi Galougahi K, Patel S, Shlofmitz RA, et al. Calcific Plaque Modification by Acoustic Shockwaves - Intravascular Lithotripsy in Coronary Interventions. Circ Cardiovasc Interventions 2021;14(1):e009354.
12. Ali ZA, Nef H, Escaned J, et al. Safety and effectiveness of coronary intravascular lithotripsy for treatment of severely calcified coronary stenoses: the disrupt CAD II study. Circ Cardiovasc Interv 2019; 12(10):e008434.
13. Genereux P, Lee AC, Kim CY, et al. Orbital Atherectomy for Treating De Novo Severely Calcified Coronary Narrowing (1-Year Results from the Pivotal ORBIT II Trial). Am J Cardiol 2015;115(12):1685–90.
14. Redfors B, Sharma SK, Saito S, et al. Novel micro crown orbital atherectomy for severe lesion

calcification: coronary orbital atherectomy system study (COAST). Circ Cardiovasc Interv 2020;13(8): e008993.

15. Karimi Galougahi K, Shlofmitz RA, Ben-Yehuda O, et al. Guiding light: insights into atherectomy by optical coherence tomography. JACC Cardiovasc Interv 2016;9(22):2362–3.

16. Gohbara M, Sugano T, Matsumoto Y, et al. Is crossability of the classic crown with the glide assist superior to the micro crown in the Diamondback 360(R) coronary orbital atherectomy system? Cardiovasc Interv Ther 2020;35(4):361–70.

17. Shlofmitz E, Martinsen BJ, Lee M, et al. Orbital atherectomy for the treatment of severely calcified coronary lesions: evidence, technique, and best practices. Expert Rev Med Devices 2017;14(11): 867–79.

18. Tomey MI, Sharma SK. Interventional options for coronary artery calcification. Curr Cardiol Rep 2016;18(2):12.

19. Koster R, Kahler J, Brockhoff C, et al. Laser coronary angioplasty: history, present and future. Am J Cardiovasc Drugs 2002;2(3):197–207.

20. Ambrosini V, Sorropago G, Laurenzano E, et al. Early outcome of high energy Laser (Excimer) facilitated coronary angioplasty ON hARD and complex calcified and balloOn-resistant coronary lesions: LEONARDO Study. Cardiovasc Revasc Med 2015;16(3):141–6.

21. Ashikaga T, Yoshikawa S, Isobe M. The effectiveness of excimer laser coronary atherectomy with contrast medium for underexpanded stent: The findings of optical frequency domain imaging. Catheter Cardiovasc Interv 2015;86(5):946–9.

22. Yin D, Maehara A, Mezzafonte S, et al. Excimer laser angioplasty-facilitated fracturing of napkin-ring peri-stent calcium in a chronically underexpanded stent: documentation by optical coherence tomography. JACC Cardiovasc Interv 2015;8(8): e137–9.

23. Fernandez JP, Hobson AR, McKenzie D, et al. Beyond the balloon: excimer coronary laser atherectomy used alone or in combination with rotational atherectomy in the treatment of chronic total occlusions, non-crossable and non-expansible coronary lesions. EuroIntervention 2013;9(2):243–50.

Saphenous Vein Graft Intervention

Aditya S. Bharadwaj, MD[a], Mamas A. Mamas, BM BCh, MA, DPhil, FRCP[b],*

KEYWORDS

- Drug-eluting stent • Percutaneous coronary intervention • Restenosis • Saphenous vein graft
- Slow flow • no reflow • Embolic Protection Device

KEY POINTS

- Saphenous vein graft (SVG) interventions are associated with increased risk of periprocedural MI due to distal embolization in the short-term, and increased risk of restenosis in the long term.
- Use of embolic protection devices has been shown to decrease the risk of distal embolization and resultant no reflow and periprocedural MI.
- Direct stenting, avoiding oversizing of stents and pharmacotherapy with vasodilators are useful adjuncts in preventing slow flow and no reflow during SVG intervention.
- Meta-analysis has revealed that there is no overall difference between bare metal stents and drug eluting stents for SVG interventions.

INTRODUCTION

The first reported use of saphenous vein graft (SVG) for coronary artery bypass graft (CABG) was in 1962 by Dr Sabiston at Johns Hopkins Hospital. The surgical technique of using SVG as a bypass conduit was subsequently standardized by the Father of CABG Rene Favaloro. Six decades later, despite their inherent limitations including poor long-term patency, SVG remains the most frequently used conduit for CABG. Less than 10% of patients undergoing coronary artery bypass graft in the United States receive multiple arterial graft revascularization.[1] Historical data reveal that whereas 3% to 12% of SVGs occlude before hospital discharge, 8% to 25% fail at 1 year, and only 50% to 60% remain patent after a decade.[2–5] More recently studies have reported comparable 5-year patency of composite grafts with arterial grafts[6] and 8-year patency of SVG as high as 91%[7] due to improvement in surgical techniques and more aggressive pharmacotherapy, respectively. SVG lesions account for 5% to 10% of all percutaneous coronary interventions (PCIs).[8,9] SVG intervention is not just technically challenging but also associated with higher

short-term (periprocedural myocardial infarction [MI], in-hospital mortality), and long-term (restenosis) complications (Fig. 1).[10] In this review article the pathophysiology of SVG failure, indications for SVG intervention, technical aspects of SVG intervention, and associated complications are discussed.

PATHOPHYSIOLOGY OF SAPHENOUS VEIN GRAFT FAILURE

Early SVG failure (within a month of CABG) occurs due to acute graft thrombosis, because of technical deficiencies such as traumatic harvesting, preexisting graft pathology, or anastomotic difficulties or due to extrinsic factors such as hypercoagulability. Beyond a month, SVGs undergo a process of "arterialization" due to intimal hyperplasia, which sets in as an adaptive mechanism to the high arterial pressure. Although in most cases SVG intimal hyperplasia only causes mild luminal narrowing, it can cause significant stenosis. In the longer term, SVG intimal hyperplasia is a precursor for accelerated atherosclerosis.[1] Atherosclerosis occurring within SVGs is more aggressive and concentric compared with native

[a] Division of Cardiology, Department of Medicine, Loma Linda University Health, 11234 Anderson Street, Suite 2422, Loma Linda, CA 92354, USA; [b] Keele Cardiovascular Research Group, Centre for Prognosis Research, Institute for Primary Care and Health Sciences, Keele University, Staffordshire ST5 5BG, UK
* Corresponding author.
E-mail address: mamasmamas1@yahoo.co.uk

Intervent Cardiol Clin 11 (2022) 383–391
https://doi.org/10.1016/j.iccl.2022.05.001
2211-7458/22/© 2022 Elsevier Inc. All rights reserved.

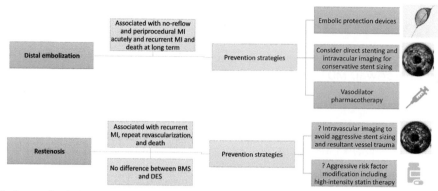

Fig. 1. Challenges for SVG intervention.

coronary atherosclerosis. Atherosclerosis within SVG also tends to be more diffuse and with thin or even absent fibrous caps making it more prone to rupture and causing acute coronary syndrome.[11] These pathophysiologic features of SVG atherosclerosis have significant technical and clinical implications. The friable and thrombotic atherosclerotic debris present within the SVG can embolize into the distal coronary bed leading to slow flow, no reflow, and periprocedural MI associated with increased mortality.[12] In addition, accelerated progression of atherosclerosis within and outside of the stented segment can result in higher rates of target lesion revascularization (TLR).

INDICATIONS FOR SAPHENOUS VEIN GRAFT INTERVENTION

SVG intervention should be performed as clinically indicated based on the presentation, patient's symptoms, and angiographic evidence of severe stenosis. Redo CABG is associated with high mortality[13] and is recommended only in situations involving multiple graft failures with potential for using the internal mammary artery for grafting and the presence of favorable native targets.[14] Anatomic or physiologic assessment of SVG lesions to determine significance, as an indication for PCI, has not been well established. Given that atherosclerosis progresses rapidly within SVGs, the role of preemptive PCI in angiographically intermediate lesions has been evaluated. The VELETI (Moderate Vein Graft Lesion Stenting with the Taxus Stent and Intravascular Ultrasound) pilot study included 57 patients with angiographically intermediate lesions (30%–60% diameter stenosis) and randomized them to PCI with paclitaxel-eluting stent or medical therapy alone. At 5 years, the PCI group had lower numerical major adverse cardiac events (MACE) (17% vs 33%, $P = .146$) and a lower statistically significant TLR (13% vs 33%, $P = .072$).[15]

This hypothesis-generating study led to the larger VELETI II trial (125 patients) with a median follow-up of 3.4 years, which demonstrated that there was no significant difference in MACE related to the target SVG lesion (10% vs 17%, $P = .21$), between PCI with drug-eluting stent (DES) and medical therapy. The investigators ascribed the lack of benefit of PCI to the occurrence of late in-stent restenosis, which negated the potential early benefits of "sealing" of an intermediate SVG lesion.[16]

In case of SVG failure, PCI can be considered to the SVG lesion or the native coronary artery depending on patient presentation, complexity of the native disease, and experience of the operator. Even though there are no randomized trial data demonstrating the superiority of native coronary PCI over SVG intervention, there are observational data suggesting better short-term and long-term outcomes with native vessel PCI,[8,17] although this is not consistent with other studies showing no differences, particularly when the native vessel is a chronic total occlusion (CTO).[18] Native coronary lesions tend to be more calcified and chronically occluded, and it is not feasible to be intervened upon in an ad hoc fashion in cases of acute coronary syndrome (ACS) presentation due to SVG failure. Previous analyses have suggested that in the context of ACS, SVG intervention is associated with worse outcomes that are likely driven by the worse clinical characteristics in patients with prior CABG.[19] Nevertheless, once these are adjusted for, clinical outcomes are similar to those who have PCI of native vessels, suggesting that it is prudent to intervene upon the SVG lesion acutely in these situations where feasible.

CHALLENGES OF SAPHENOUS VEIN GRAFT INTERVENTION

Slow flow and no reflow due to distal embolization of friable thrombotic and atheromatous debris are significant complications of SVG intervention. The incidence varies from 3.4% to 18.5% but remains significantly higher than native vessel PCI.[17] Distal embolization acutely causes chest pain, ischemic ST changes, and periprocedural MI. In the longer term, patients who develop no reflow during SVG intervention are at significantly higher risk of reinfarction and death.[20,21] In a multivariate analysis of 1056 patients undergoing SVG intervention, major creatinine kinase MB (CK-MB) elevation was the strongest independent predictor of 1-year mortality.[21] Even though distal embolization is difficult to predict, certain findings on intravascular ultrasound (IVUS) such as the presence of intraluminal mass, multiple plaque ruptures, and degenerated SVGs have been shown to be independent predictors of no reflow.[20] As discussed later, use of embolic protection devices (EPDs), direct stenting, conservative stent sizing, and vasodilator therapy have been shown to decrease the incidence or treat no reflow. Other challenges of SVG intervention include prolonged procedure time, higher radiation doses, increased contrast volume, and possibly greater risk of contrast-induced nephropathy.[22,23] In the longer term, SVG PCI is associated with high risk of restenosis irrespective of the use of bare metal stent (BMS) or DES.[22] Female sex[24] and presence of renal insufficiency[25] are independent predictors of poor short- and long-term outcomes following SVG intervention.

TECHNICAL ASPECTS OF SAPHENOUS VEIN GRAFT INTERVENTION

Stent Type: Bare Metal Stent versus Drug-Eluting Stent

Numerous randomized controlled trials (RCTs) comparing BMS versus DES for the treatment of SVG stenosis have shown inconsistent results (Table 1). A meta-analysis of 6 RCTs evaluating DES versus BMS demonstrated that there was no statistically significant difference in all-cause mortality (risk ratio [RR],1.11; 95% confidence interval [CI], 0.0.77 to 1.62; $P = .57$), cardiovascular mortality (RR, 1.00; 95% CI, 0.64–1.57; $P = .99$), MACE (RR, 0.83; 95% CI, 0.63–1.10; $P = 20$), target vessel revascularization (RR, 0.73; 95% CI, 0.48–1.11; $P = .14$), MI (RR, 0.74; 95% CI, 0.48–1.16; $P = .19$), or stent thrombosis (RR, 1.06; 95% CI, 0.42–2.65; $P = .90$). The most recent RCT also included in the aforementioned meta-analysis was the DIVA trial, which used second-generation DES in the vast majority in the DES arm with a median 2.7-year follow-up; it also revealed similar

rates of target vessel failure.[26] Covered stents made of polytetrafluoroethylene in theory may decrease distal embolization by trapping friable debris against the SVG wall and prevent restenosis by creating a barrier for smooth muscle hyperplasia. However, these theoretic benefits did not translate into clinical benefits as demonstrated by prospective randomized trials.[27–29]

Embolic Protection Devices

The use of EPD during SVG intervention is a class I recommendation by the American College of Cardiology Foundation/American Heart Association Task Force on Practice Guidelines and the Society for Cardiovascular Angiography and Interventions guidelines. Despite their class I recommendation, EPDs are used only in 21% of SVG interventions likely due to technical challenges and the associated time and cost.[30] There are 2 main categories of EPDs as described in the following paragraphs and in Table 2.

Distal balloon occlusion device allows inflation of a balloon distally thereby creating a static column of blood and preventing distal embolization. At the end of the intervention, the column of blood along with the trapped debris is aspirated before deflation of the balloon. Advantages of distal balloon occlusion device include low crossing profile and the ability to trap particles of all sizes including neurohormonal mediators such as serotonin and thromboxane, which have adverse effects on distal microvasculature and are released due to SVG manipulation. Disadvantages include ischemia caused by occlusion of blood flow within the SVG, inability to fully aspirate the column of debris-laden blood, and potential injury to the SVG endothelium at the site of balloon inflation. The PercuSurge GuardWire (Medtronic, Minneapolis, MN, USA) is a Food and Drug Administration (FDA)-approved distal balloon occlusion device. The SAFER (Saphenous Vein Graft Angioplasty Free of Emboli, Randomized) RCT compared the PercuSurge GuardWire with a conventional guidewire and demonstrated a 42% relative reduction in MACE, which was primarily driven by MI (8.6% vs 14.7%, $P = .008$) and no-reflow phenomenon (3% vs 9%, $P = .02$).[31]

Distal embolic filters are used to trap debris that embolize during SVG intervention.

Table 1
Summary of select larger (N > 100) contemporary trials comparing bare metal stents versus drug-eluting stents for saphenous vein graft intervention

Trial Name, Year	Number of Patients	Type of Stent Used	Percentage of EPD Use	Primary End Point	Duration of Follow-up	Result
ISAR-CABG, 2011[44]	610	DES: permanent polymer paclitaxel and sirolimus-eluting stent, biodegradable polymer sirolimus-eluting stent BMS: Multilink vision (Abbott Vascular, Santa Clara, CA, USA), Driver stent (Medtronic, Santa Rosa CA, USA), Yukon stent (Translumina, Hechingen, Germany)	< 5%	Composite of death, MI, and TLR	12 mo	DES reduced incidence of primary end point compared with BMS (15% vs 22%, P = .02)
ISAR-CABG 5-y outcomes, 2018[45]	610	Same as mentioned above	< 5%	Composite of death, MI, and TLR	60 mo	At 5-y follow up there was no difference in primary end point between DES and BMS groups (55.5% vs 53.6%, P = .89)
BASKET SAVAGE, 2016[46]	173	DES: Paclitaxel-eluting Taxus Liberte (Boston Scientific, Natick, MA, USA) BMS: Liberte (Boston Scientific, Natick, MA, USA)	66%	Composite of cardiac death, MI, and TVR	36 mo	DES associated with lower incidence of primary end point compared with BMS (12.4% vs 29.8%, P = .0012)
DIVA, 2018	597	DES: 93% second-generation, 7% first-generation DES BMS: contemporary BMS	BMS group: 69% DES group: 68%	Composite of cardiac death, target vessel MI, and TVR	2.7 y	No difference between DES and BMS (37% vs 34%, P = .44)

Table 2
Table summarizing types of embolic protection devices

Type of EPD	Commonly Used Commercially Available Devices	Advantages	Disadvantages	Data Supporting Use
Distal balloon occlusion device	PercuSurge GuardWire (Medtronic, Minneapolis, MN, USA)	Small crossing profile, able to trap debris of all sizes as well as neurohormonal mediators such as serotonin and thromboxane, which are released during SVG intervention and cause adverse effects to distal microvasculature	Ischemia caused by occlusion of blood flow, inability to fully aspirate column of debris-laden blood, requires a 30-mm distal landing zone for deployment	SAFER trial: GuardWire was better than conventional guidewire with 42% relative reduction in MACE, driven by MI (8.6% vs 14.7%, $P = .008$) and no reflow (3% vs 9%, $P = .02$)
Distal protection filter	FilterWireEZ (Boston Scientific, Natick, MA, USA); SpiderFx (Medtronic, Santa Rosa, CA, USA)	Relatively easy to use, maintains perfusion during intervention, especially important in unstable patients	May not cross tight stenosis, requires a 30-mm distal landing zone for deployment	• FIRE Trial: FilterWire was noninferior to GuardWire, 30-d MACE rates (9.9% vs 11.6%; $P = .0008$ for noninferiority) • SPIDER Trial: Spider FX was noninferior to FilterWireEZ or GuardWire, 30-d MACE rates (9.1% vs 8.4%; $P = .01$)

These filters are sheathed within a catheter, delivered over a guidewire, and deployed distal to the SVG lesion. At the end of the procedure, they are retrieved by the catheter along with retained debris. These filters are relatively easy to use and allow for continued perfusion of the distal coronary bed unlike occlusion devices, thereby having a distinct advantage in hemodynamically unstable patients, left ventricular dysfunction, and interventions on the last remaining conduit.[10] The 2 most commonly used embolic protection filters are FilterWireEZ (Boston Scientific, Natick, MA, USA) and the SpiderFx (Medtronic, Santa Rosa, CA, USA). FilterWireEZ was compared with the GuardWire distal balloon occlusion and aspiration system, in the randomized FIRE trial, which included 651 patients.[32] FilterWireEZ was found to be noninferior to GuardWire system and had comparable 30-day MACE rates (9.9% vs 11.6%; $P = .0008$ for noninferiority). Similarly, the SpiderFx filter was compared with FilterWireEZ or GuardWire system in the SPIDER randomized trial. The trial reported noninferior ($P = .012$) 30-day MACE rates of SpiderFx (9.1) compared with either FilterWireEZ or GuardWire (8.4).[33]

It is to be noted that both the distal occlusion balloon and the distal embolic filter devices require at least a 30-mm relatively disease-free "landing zone" proximal to the graft anastomosis for their use.

Excimer Laser Coronary Angioplasty

ECLA is FDA approved for the treatment of thrombotic SVG lesions, although there are no guidelines regarding its use owing to the lack of randomized data. Conceptually ECLA causes "vaporization" of thrombotic, friable atherosclerotic plaque present in SVG lesions and may reduce the risk of distal embolization. A prospective case control registry with patients with non-ST elevation MI with SVG culprit lesions compared patients undergoing SVG intervention with ECLA versus EPD (FilterWireEZ and the SpiderFx). The investigators reported a lower incidence of angiographic microvascular obstruction (13% vs 32%, $P = .09$) and type IVa MI (21% vs 49%, $P = .04$) in the ECLA group compared with the EPD group.[34]

Consideration for Direct Stenting

Avoiding predilation of SVG lesions may potentially reduce the incidence of distal embolization and the resultant slow-flow or no-reflow phenomenon. Direct stenting of SVG lesions may trap debris against the vessel wall and cause less SVG wall trauma. In a study of 527 consecutive patients undergoing SVG intervention, direct stenting was associated with lower CK-MB release periprocedurally and lower TLR at 1 year compared with a conventional stenting.[35] A posthoc analysis of patients in the DIVA trial comparing direct stenting (without predilation or postdilation) with "balloon stent" strategy demonstrated a lower incidence of definite stent thrombosis (1% vs 5%, $P = .009$), definite/probable stent thrombosis (5% vs 11%, $P = .009$), and target vessel MI (8% vs 14%, $P = .023$) in the direct stenting group at long-term follow-up (median 2.7 years).[36] However, in our experience predilation of SVG lesions is inevitable in certain situation such as the presence of severe calcification and in-stent restenosis due to a previously underexpanded stent.

Stent Sizing

The strategy of undersizing stents in SVGs has been proposed as a possible mechanism to reduce distal embolization as well as vessel wall trauma. Two intravascular imaging-guided studies have demonstrated a lower incidence of periprocedural MI without any long-term difference in TLR with the strategy of undersizing stents. Hong and colleagues[37] used the ratio of stent diameter to average reference lumen diameter based on IVUS and divided patients into 3 groups (ratio of <0.89, 0.9–1.0, and > 1.0). The group with most conservative stent sizing (<0.89) had the lowest amount of plaque intrusion and lowest risk of CK-MB elevation without any significant differences in 1-year TLR or target vessel revascularization (TVR).[37] Likewise, Iakovou and colleagues[38] used IVUS-derived ratios of final stent cross-sectional area to reference lumen cross-sectional area to demonstrate that more aggressive stent expansion was associated with higher in-hospital non-Q wave MI, any MI at 1-year follow-up with no improvement in TVR at 1 year. It is, nevertheless, important to not conflate undersizing with malapposition, which would be associated with an increased risk of stent thrombosis in these settings.

Periprocedural Vasodilator Pharmacotherapy

Vasodilators such as adenosine, nitroprusside, verapamil, and nicardipine are typically used during SVG intervention to treat slow flow or no-reflow phenomenon. Sdringola and colleagues[39] in a retrospective study of 143 patients reported that preemptive intragraft administration of adenosine does not prevent slow flow. However, rapid and high-dose administration of intragraft adenosine ($\geq$5 boluses of 24 µg each) was successful in treating slow flow/no-reflow situation. Adenosine has the potential to cause severe bradycardia due to its effect on the sinoatrial and atrioventricular node. However, it is transient owing to its short half-life. In a small RCT, pretreatment with intragraft verapamil was shown to prevent no reflow and was associated with a trend toward improved myocardial flow.[40] In case of slow flow/no reflow intragraft administration of nitroprusside has been shown to rapidly and significantly improve distal coronary flow.[41] Verapamil may cause hypotension in patients with severe left ventricular dysfunction, whereas nitroprusside tends to cause hypotension in those with volume depletion. Nicardipine is a potent arteriolar dilator with less propensity to cause hypotension and has also been shown to be very effective in preventing and treating no reflow during SVG intervention.[42]

SUMMARY

SVGs are intrinsically more prone to accelerated atherosclerosis compared with native coronary arteries. SVG intervention poses several challenges both in the short term and long term. Distal embolization during SVG intervention results in no reflow and periprocedural MI, which is in turn a predictor of reinfarction and late mortality. EPDs should be used to mitigate these risks, and consideration must be given for direct stenting. Intragraft vasodilators are a useful adjunct in the prevention and treatment of no reflow. Intravascular imaging is a vital tool to understand lesion characteristics and determine vessel diameter so as to prevent oversizing of stents. SVG interventions are associated with high restenosis rates with no differences in clinical outcomes between BMSs and DESs, although the authors would advocate using second-generation DESs, which have been shown to have superior outcomes in SCG lesions compared with first-generation DESs and BMSs.[43]

CLINICS CARE POINTS

- When performing SVG interventions it is recommended to use an embolic protection device when technically feasible, in order to avoid distal embolization and its resultant periprocedural MI.

- Consider direct stenting of SVG lesions and intravascular imaging to avoid oversizing of stents during SVG intervention to decrease the incidence of distal embolization.

- Pharmacotherapy with vasodilators delivered through the guide catheter may be of adjunctive benefit in decreasing the occurrence of slow flow and no-reflow following SVG intervention.

REFERENCES

1. Xenogiannis I, Zenati M, Bhatt DL, et al. Saphenous Vein Graft Failure: From Pathophysiology to Prevention and Treatment Strategies. Circulation 2021;144(9):728–45.
2. Goldman S, Zadina K, Moritz T, et al. Long-term patency of saphenous vein and left internal mammary artery grafts after coronary artery bypass surgery: results from a Department of Veterans Affairs Cooperative Study. J Am Coll Cardiol 2004;44(11):2149–56.
3. Lopes RD, Hafley GE, Allen KB, et al. Endoscopic versus open vein-graft harvesting in coronary-artery bypass surgery. N Engl J Med 2009;361(3):235–44.
4. Magee MJ, Alexander JH, Hafley G, et al. Coronary artery bypass graft failure after on-pump and off-pump coronary artery bypass: findings from PREVENT IV. Ann Thorac Surg 2008;85(2):494–9 [discussion: 499–500].
5. Zhao DX, Leacche M, Balaguer JM, et al. Routine intraoperative completion angiography after coronary artery bypass grafting and 1-stop hybrid revascularization results from a fully integrated hybrid catheterization laboratory/operating room. J Am Coll Cardiol 2009;53(3):232–41.
6. Kim MS, Hwang HY, Kim JS, et al. Saphenous vein versus right internal thoracic artery as a Y-composite graft: Five-year angiographic and clinical results of a randomized trial. J Thorac Cardiovasc Surg 2018;156(4):1424–33.e1.
7. Hage A, Voisine P, Erthal F, et al. Eight-year follow-up of the Clopidogrel After Surgery for Coronary Artery Disease (CASCADE) trial. J Thorac Cardiovasc Surg 2018;155(1):212–222 e212.
8. Brilakis ES, Rao SV, Banerjee S, et al. Percutaneous coronary intervention in native arteries versus bypass grafts in prior coronary artery bypass grafting patients: a report from the National Cardiovascular Data Registry. JACC Cardiovasc Interv 2011;4(8):844–50.
9. Brodie BR, Wilson H, Stuckey T, et al. Outcomes with drug-eluting versus bare-metal stents in saphenous vein graft intervention results from the STENT (strategic transcatheter evaluation of new

therapies) group. JACC Cardiovasc Interv 2009; 2(11):1105–12.

10. Lee MS, Park SJ, Kandzari DE, et al. Saphenous vein graft intervention. JACC Cardiovasc Interv 2011; 4(8):831–43.

11. Yazdani SK, Farb A, Nakano M, et al. Pathology of drug-eluting versus bare-metal stents in saphenous vein bypass graft lesions. JACC Cardiovasc Interv 2012;5(6):666–74.

12. O'Connor GT, Malenka DJ, Quinton H, et al. Multivariate prediction of in-hospital mortality after percutaneous coronary interventions in 1994-1996. Northern New England Cardiovascular Disease Study Group. J Am Coll Cardiol 1999;34(3):681–91.

13. Mohamed MO, Shoaib A, Gogas B, et al. Trends of repeat revascularization choice in patients with prior coronary artery bypass surgery. Catheter Cardiovasc Interv 2021;98(3):470–80.

14. Sousa-Uva M, Neumann FJ, Ahlsson A, et al. 2018 ESC/EACTS Guidelines on myocardial revascularization. Eur J Cardiothorac Surg 2019;55(1):4–90.

15. Rodes-Cabau J, Bertrand OF, Larose E, et al. Five-year follow-up of the plaque sealing with paclitaxel-eluting stents vs medical therapy for the treatment of intermediate nonobstructive saphenous vein graft lesions (VELETI) trial. Can J Cardiol 2014; 30(1):138–45.

16. Rodes-Cabau J, Jolly SS, Cairns J, et al. Sealing Intermediate Nonobstructive Coronary Saphenous Vein Graft Lesions With Drug-Eluting Stents as a New Approach to Reducing Cardiac Events: A Randomized Controlled Trial. Circ Cardiovasc Interv 2016;9(11):e004336.

17. Brilakis ES, O'Donnell CI, Penny W, et al. Percutaneous Coronary Intervention in Native Coronary Arteries Versus Bypass Grafts in Patients With Prior Coronary Artery Bypass Graft Surgery: Insights From the Veterans Affairs Clinical Assessment, Reporting, and Tracking Program. JACC Cardiovasc Interv 2016;9(9):884–93.

18. Shoaib A, Johnson TW, Banning A, et al. Clinical Outcomes of Percutaneous Coronary Intervention for Chronic Total Occlusion in Native Coronary Arteries vs Saphenous Vein Grafts. J Invasive Cardiol 2020;32(9):350–7.

19. Shoaib A, Kinnaird T, Curzen N, et al. Outcomes Following Percutaneous Coronary Intervention in Non-ST-Segment-Elevation Myocardial Infarction Patients With Coronary Artery Bypass Grafts. Circ Cardiovasc Interv 2018;11(11):e006824.

20. Hong YJ, Jeong MH, Ahn Y, et al. Intravascular ultrasound findings that are predictive of no reflow after percutaneous coronary intervention for saphenous vein graft disease. Am J Cardiol 2012;109(11): 1576–81.

21. Hong MK, Mehran R, Dangas G, et al. Creatine kinase-MB enzyme elevation following successful

saphenous vein graft intervention is associated with late mortality. Circulation 1999;100(24):2400–5.

22. Xenogiannis I, Tajti P, Hall AB, et al. Update on Cardiac Catheterization in Patients With Prior Coronary Artery Bypass Graft Surgery. JACC Cardiovasc Interv 2019;12(17):1635–49.

23. Teramoto T, Tsuchikane E, Matsuo H, et al. Initial success rate of percutaneous coronary intervention for chronic total occlusion in a native coronary artery is decreased in patients who underwent previous coronary artery bypass graft surgery. JACC Cardiovasc Interv 2014;7(1):39–46.

24. Ahmed JM, Dangas G, Lansky AJ, et al. Influence of gender on early and one-year clinical outcomes after saphenous vein graft stenting. Am J Cardiol 2001;87(4):401–5.

25. Lee MS, Hu PP, Aragon J, et al. Impact of chronic renal insufficiency on clinical outcomes in patients undergoing saphenous vein graft intervention with drug-eluting stents: a multicenter Southern Californian Registry. Catheter Cardiovasc Interv 2010;76(2):272–8.

26. Brilakis ES, Edson R, Bhatt DL, et al. Drug-eluting stents versus bare-metal stents in saphenous vein grafts: a double-blind, randomised trial. Lancet 2018;391(10134):1997–2007.

27. Turco MA, Buchbinder M, Popma JJ, et al. Pivotal, randomized U.S. study of the Symbiottrade mark covered stent system in patients with saphenous vein graft disease: eight-month angiographic and clinical results from the Symbiot III trial. Catheter Cardiovasc Interv 2006;68(3):379–88.

28. Stankovic G, Colombo A, Presbitero P, et al. Randomized evaluation of polytetrafluoroethylene-covered stent in saphenous vein grafts: the Randomized Evaluation of polytetrafluoroethylene COVERed stent in Saphenous vein grafts (RECOVERS) Trial. Circulation 2003;108(1):37–42.

29. Stone GW, Goldberg S, O'Shaughnessy C, et al. 5-year follow-up of polytetrafluoroethylene-covered stents compared with bare-metal stents in aorto-coronary saphenous vein grafts the randomized BARRICADE (barrier approach to restenosis: restrict intima to curtail adverse events) trial. JACC Cardiovasc Interv 2011;4(3):300–9.

30. Levine GN, Bates ER, Blankenship JC, et al. 2011 ACCF/AHA/SCAI Guideline for Percutaneous Coronary Intervention: a report of the American College of Cardiology Foundation/American Heart Association Task Force on Practice Guidelines and the Society for Cardiovascular Angiography and Interventions. Circulation 2011;124(23):e574–651.

31. Baim DS, Wahr D, George B, et al. Randomized trial of a distal embolic protection device during percutaneous intervention of saphenous vein aorto-coronary bypass grafts. Circulation 2002; 105(11):1285–90.

32. Stone GW, Rogers C, Hermiller J, et al. Randomized comparison of distal protection with a filter-based catheter and a balloon occlusion and aspiration system during percutaneous intervention of diseased saphenous vein aorto-coronary bypass grafts. Circulation 2003;108(5):548–53.

33. Dixon SR, O'Neill W, Investigators S. Saphenous vein graft protection in a distal embolic protection randomized trial. Transcatheter Cardiovascular Therapeutics. 2005.

34. Niccoli G, Belloni F, Cosentino N, et al. Case-control registry of excimer laser coronary angioplasty versus distal protection devices in patients with acute coronary syndromes due to saphenous vein graft disease. Am J Cardiol 2013;112(10):1586–91.

35. Leborgne L, Cheneau E, Pichard A, et al. Effect of direct stenting on clinical outcome in patients treated with percutaneous coronary intervention on saphenous vein graft. Am Heart J 2003;146(3):501–6.

36. Latif F, Uyeda L, Edson R, et al. Stent-Only Versus Adjunctive Balloon Angioplasty Approach for Saphenous Vein Graft Percutaneous Coronary Intervention: Insights From DIVA Trial. Circ Cardiovasc Interv 2020;13(2):e008494.

37. Hong YJ, Pichard AD, Mintz GS, et al. Outcome of undersized drug-eluting stents for percutaneous coronary intervention of saphenous vein graft lesions. Am J Cardiol 2010;105(2):179–85.

38. Iakovou I, Dangas G, Mintz GS, et al. Relation of final lumen dimensions in saphenous vein grafts after stent implantation to outcome. Am J Cardiol 2004;93(8):963–8.

39. Sdringola S, Assali A, Ghani M, et al. Adenosine use during aortocoronary vein graft interventions reverses but does not prevent the slow-no reflow phenomenon. Catheter Cardiovasc Interv 2000;51(4):394–9.

40. Michaels AD, Appleby M, Otten MH, et al. Pretreatment with intragraft verapamil prior to percutaneous coronary intervention of saphenous vein graft lesions: results of the randomized, controlled vasodilator prevention on no-reflow (VAPOR) trial. J Invasive Cardiol 2002;14(6):299–302.

41. Hillegass WB, Dean NA, Liao L, et al. Treatment of no-reflow and impaired flow with the nitric oxide donor nitroprusside following percutaneous coronary interventions: initial human clinical experience. J Am Coll Cardiol 2001;37(5):1335–43.

42. Fischell TA, Subraya RG, Ashraf K, et al. Pharmacologic" distal protection using prophylactic, intragraft nicardipine to prevent no-reflow and non-Q-wave myocardial infarction during elective saphenous vein graft intervention. J Invasive Cardiol 2007;19(2):58–62.

43. Iqbal J, Kwok CS, Kontopantelis E, et al. Choice of Stent for Percutaneous Coronary Intervention of Saphenous Vein Grafts. Circ Cardiovasc Interv 2017;10(4):e004457.

44. Mehilli J, Pache J, Abdel-Wahab M, et al. Drug-eluting versus bare-metal stents in saphenous vein graft lesions (ISAR-CABG): a randomised controlled superiority trial. Lancet 2011;378(9796):1071–8.

45. Colleran R, Kufner S, Mehilli J, et al. Efficacy Over Time With Drug-Eluting Stents in Saphenous Vein Graft Lesions. J Am Coll Cardiol 2018;71(18):1973–82.

46. Fahrni G, Farah A, Engstrom T, et al. Long-Term Results After Drug-Eluting Versus Bare-Metal Stent Implantation in Saphenous Vein Grafts: Randomized Controlled Trial. J Am Heart Assoc 2020;9(20):e017434.

Intravascular Lithotripsy for Treatment of Calcified Coronary Artery Disease

Dean J. Kereiakes, MD, MSCAI[a],*, Ziad A. Ali, MD, DPhil[b],
Robert F. Riley, MD[a], Timothy D. Smith, MD[a],
Richard A. Shlofmitz, MD[c]

KEYWORDS

- Coronary calcification • Coronary revascularization • Coronary stents
- Percutaneous coronary intervention • Calcium modification

KEY POINTS

- Severe coronary calcification increases procedural complications and adverse clinical outcomes after percutaneous coronary intervention.
- Intravascular lithotripsy (IVL) is a novel technique that uses acoustic shock waves in a balloon delivery system to induce fractures in coronary calcium, which facilitate stent expansion and luminal gain.
- The Disrupt CAD I to IV clinical trials demonstrate the safety and effectiveness of lesion preparation with IVL to optimize coronary stent implantation in severely calcified vessels.

INTRODUCTION

Advanced age and an increasing frequency of diabetes mellitus, systemic hypertension, and chronic kidney disease contribute to the increasing prevalence in severity of coronary calcification.[1,2] Calcified coronary plaque negatively impacts angiographic and clinical outcomes following percutaneous coronary intervention (PCI) by impeding stent delivery, causing delamination of polymer with alteration of drug elution kinetics, and is associated with stent asymmetry, malapposition, and underexpansion.[3–5] Suboptimal stent expansion is the strongest predictor of subsequent stent thrombosis or restenosis.[6,7] Despite the use of high-pressure, noncompliant balloon catheters, cutting/scoring balloons, and atheroablative technologies (laser, rotational or orbital atherectomy) to modify coronary calcium,[8,9] PCI of heavily calcified lesions is more often associated with both early (coronary dissection, vessel perforation, myocardial infarction [MI]) and late (restenosis, stent thrombosis, repeat vascularization) adverse events. Indeed, the presence of severe target lesion calcification portends adverse outcomes in the periprocedural, early (PCI procedure to 30 days), late (30 days to 1 year), and very late (>1 year) periods when compared with PCI without severe lesion calcification.[7,10–13] Both to 1 year and beyond, the occurrence of cardiac death, MI, or repeat coronary revascularization is increased following PCI with the presence of severe target lesion calcification. Although atheroablation may facilitate stent delivery and expansion, the extent of calcium modification is limited by guidewire bias and may be associated with periprocedural complications including slow or no reflow, coronary dissection, perforation, and MI.[8,9,14,15] These complications are more frequent following atherectomy compared with balloon-based therapies. Furthermore, the eccentricity of ablation effect on calcium modification may have limited

---

[a] The Carl and Edyth Lindner Center for Research and Education at The Christ Hospital, 2123 Auburn Avenue Suite 424, Cincinnati, OH 45219, USA; [b] Columbia University Medical Center, 622 W 168th Street, New York, NY 10032, USA; [c] St. Francis Hospital & Heart Center, 100 Port Washington Boulevard Suite 105, Roslyn, NY 11576, USA
* Corresponding author.
E-mail address: Dean.Kereiakes@thechristhospital.com

Intervent Cardiol Clin 11 (2022) 393–404
https://doi.org/10.1016/j.iccl.2022.02.004
2211-7458/22/© 2022 Elsevier Inc. All rights reserved.

impact on deep calcium so that stent expansion remains constrained.[14–16] High-pressure noncompliant balloon dilation may have insufficient force to modify concentric, circumferential calcium, whereas balloon dilation may be biased toward noncalcified arterial segments in the presence of eccentric calcification with consequent dissection at the fibrocalcific interface rather than true calcium modification.[16] Intravascular lithotripsy (IVL) incorporates principles used to transmit acoustic energy for the treatment of nephrolithiasis (ie, extracorporeal lithotripsy) (Fig. 1).[17] IVL has been evaluated as an adjunct to coronary stenting in 4 single-arm, nonrandomized studies (Table 1), which have collectively and uniformly demonstrated high rates of device and procedural success with excellent early angiographic and clinical outcomes.[16,18–20] These studies have provided evidence for device safety and effectiveness as well as insights into the mechanisms of calcium modification. Each study incorporated an intravascular imaging substudy using optical coherent tomography (OCT) with independent OCT core laboratory adjudication.

DISCUSSION

Intravascular Imaging in the Evaluation of Treatment of Coronary Calcification

The presence, extent, and distribution of coronary calcium as demonstrated by intravascular imaging provide prognostic information that may be useful to inform PCI strategy. Although calcium is often defined radiographically as radiopacities without cardiac motion, before contrast injection, generally on both sides of the arterial lumen, intravascular imaging provides more sensitive and specific information.[21,22] Indeed, 30% to 50% of calcified plaque goes undetected by radiographic imaging alone. Compared with intravascular ultrasonography, OCT imaging is more accurate in defining the presence and extent of deep calcium and for reliably providing quantitative indices.[23] The greater the calcium arc or angle, length, or thickness of calcium, the greater the likelihood of subsequent stent under expansion.[24,25] These quantitative measures (calcium arc, length, thickness) have been incorporated into a scoring system (calcium volume index [CVI] score) to predict stent under expansion and to inform therapeutic strategy. The CVI score assigns 2 points for calcium arc greater than 180°, 1 point for calcium length greater than 5.0 mm, and 1 point for calcium thickness greater than 0.5 mm. A score of 4 is associated with a high rate of subsequent stent under expansion (≥80%) without the use of adjunctive calcium

modified technologies. During coronary OCT imaging, calcium is defined as superficial if the luminal leading edge of calcium is located within 0.5 mm from the surface of plaque.[16] These quantitative baseline (before PCI) measures have been incorporated into a therapeutic algorithm to guide PCI of moderate to severely calcified coronary lesions or if inadequate balloon expansion is observed during target lesion preparation.[26] A target lesion CVI score less than 4.0 may be approached with noncompliant or cutting/scoring balloons with atheroablative technologies reserved for balloon therapy failures. Intravascular imaging provides a more exact method for determining accurate vessel size as well as optimal IVL balloon and stent sizing. Furthermore, OCT can be performed following the use of calcium-modifying technologies to determine adequacy of affect as well as after stent deployment to evaluate the adequacy of stent apposition and expansion, minimum stent area (MSA), and stent edge assessment for dissection for residual plaque burden. OCT has also been used to guide IVL pulse management with respect to balloon/emitter repositioning as well as the delivery of more pulses if calcium fractures are not visualized (Richard Shlofmitz, personal communication, 2021).

Intravascular Lithotripsy Mechanisms of Action

Modification of sonic pressure waves from extracorporeal shockwave lithotripsy to intravascular lithotripsy

Vascular calcium poses unique challenges that necessitate adaptations of extracorporeal shockwave lithotripsy (ESWL) for safe and effective intravascular treatment. These modifications include (1) transition from focused to unfocused energy, (2) reduction in overall energy, (3) minimizing peak negative pressure pulses, (4) encapsulation within a fluid-filled balloon, (5) controlled pulse frequency, and (6) arrangement of emitters in series along the shaft of the catheter to facilitate longitudinal treatment of the calcified vessel.[17]

In ESWL, a spark between 2 electrodes results in the formation of an acoustic pressure wave that expands spherically outward from the emitter. As the spark gap is initiated outside the body, the energy requirement to fracture calculi is high, and thus high-energy shockwaves are focused through parabolic reflection, concentrating the fragmenting impact on the calculi. A standard electrohydraulic (EHL) shockwave pressure pulse lasts ~5 to 10 μs and consists of a near-instantaneously developed peak

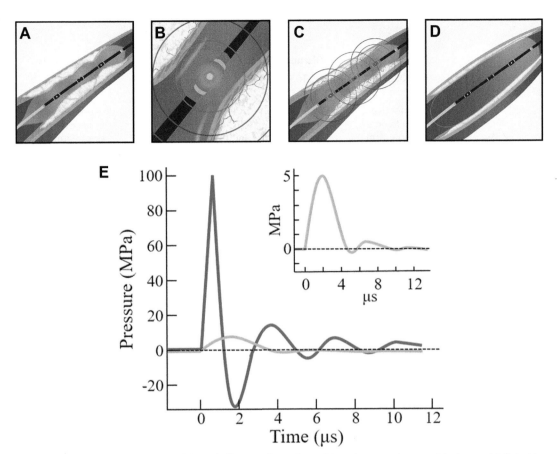

Fig. 1. IVL shockwave generation. (A) IVL balloon catheter is positioned across the target lesion and inflated to 4 atm. (B) Emitter spark gap discharge produces compressive shockwaves that emanate spherically outward; vapor bubble formation is contained with the integrated balloon. (C) IVL shockwaves affect superficial and deep calcium. (D) After IVL therapy is delivered, the balloon is inflated to 6 atm before deflation. (E) Superimposed IVL (blue) and ESWL (red) waveforms. Note the contrast in positive and negative peak pressures between the 2 EHL technologies. Representative IVL waveform demonstrating positive peak pressure of ∼5 MPa with minimal negative peak pressure generation (inset). ESWL, extracorporeal shockwave lithotripsy. (Reprinted from Kereiakes DJ, Virmani R, Hokama JY, et al. Principles of intravascular lithotripsy for calcific plaque modification. JACC Cardiovasc Interv 2021;14(12):1275–92.)

positive component of 300 to 1000 atm and negative pressure trough of 80 to 150 atm.[27] By modifying the pulse width applied to the emitters, and eliminating parabolic focusing, the IVL acoustic pressure has been significantly reduced to a positive peak pressure of ∼50 atm and near-negligible negative peak pressures (∼-0.3 MPa or -3 atm), which are safer for the intravascular space.[17] Moreover, because the goal of IVL is calcium fracture as opposed to pulverization with ESWL, these peak positive and negative pressures are appropriate for inducing vascular calcium fracture while limiting the potential for soft tissue injury associated with higher energy levels. Furthermore, because IVL shockwaves are initiated in close proximity to the target vascular calcium, much less energy is required for IVL compared with ESWL.[17]

Role of balloon in heat dissipation

The careful encapsulation of emitters in series within a fluid filled balloon serves to eliminate directional bias, mitigate thermal injury, and provide longitudinal therapy, all of which are essential elements of IVL technologies in the vascular space.[28] As the emitters are centrally placed on the balloon catheter shaft, inflation of the balloon centralizes the emitters, moving them away from the vascular wall, thus eliminating direct application of the spark to the vessel wall. When inflated to 4 atm, the minimum pressure required to fill the balloon, the temperature change within the blood vessel is less than less than 0.5° C (well below the thermal injury threshold of approximately 43° C). Indeed,[17] the centralization of the emitters within the balloon also eliminates directional bias, because

Table 1
Major characteristics of the 4 Disrupt CAD studies

	Disrupt CAD I[1]	Disrupt CAD II[2]	Disrupt CAD III[3]	Disrupt CAD IV[4]
ClinicalTrials.gov identifier	NCT02650128	NCT03328949	NCT03595176	NCT04151628
Study design	Prospective, multicenter, single arm	Prospective, multicenter, single arm	Prospective, multicenter, single arm	Prospective, multicenter, single arm
Enrollment period	December 2015–September 2016	May 2018–March 2019	January 2019–March 2020	November 2019–April 2020
Number of patients	60	120	384	64
Number of centers	7	15	47	8
Participating regions	AU, EU	EU	US, EU	Japan
Independent angiographic core laboratory assessment	Yes	Yes	Yes	Yes
Independent Clinical Events Committee adjudication	Yes	Yes	Yes	Yes
Periprocedural MI definition	CK-MB >3× ULN with or without new pathologic Q wave	CK-MB >3× ULN with or without new pathologic Q wave	CK-MB >3× ULN with or without new pathologic Q wave	CK-MB >3× ULN with or without new pathologic Q wave
Target lesions	Severely calcified, de novo coronary artery lesions	Severely calcified, de novo coronary artery lesions	Severely calcified, de novo coronary artery lesions	Severely calcified, de novo coronary artery lesions
Lesion locations	LM, LAD, RCA, LCx	LM, LAD, RCA, LCx	LM, LAD, RCA, LCx	LM, LAD, RCA, LCx
Target lesion length	≤ 32 mm	≤ 32 mm	≤ 40 mm	≤ 40 mm
Target lesion reference vessel diameter	2.5 mm–4.0 mm	2.5 mm–4.0 mm	2.5 mm–4.0 mm	2.5 mm–4.0 mm
Target lesion stenosis	≥50% and <100%	≥50% and <100%	≥70% and <100%	≥70% and <100%
30-d follow-up complete	60/60 (100%)	119/120 (99.2%)	383/384 (99.7%)	64/64 (100%)

NCT, national clinical trial; AU, Australia; EU, European Union; US, United States; LM, left main; LAD, left anterior descending; RCA, right coronary artery; LCx, left circumflex, ULN, upper limit of normal; CK-MB, creatine kinase myocardial band-isoenzyme.

Reprinted from Kereiakes DJ, Di Mario C, Riley RF, et al. Intravascular lithotripsy for treatment of calcified coronary lesions: patient-level pooled analysis of the Disrupt CAD studies. JACC Cardiovasc Interv 2021;14(12):1337–48.

the balloon acts as a scaffold, facilitating delivery of energy circumferentially, and evenly. Moreover, the pulse frequency of 1 Hz also minimizes the risk of thermal injury, because each pulse wave is completed before the next pulse, allowing dissipation of heat between pulses. After 10 pulses the IVL catheter is switched to standby mode automatically, reminding the operator to deflate the balloon and allow perfusion of blood, further dissipating even the small amount of heat that is generated during IVL therapy.[29] Finally, the placement of electrodes in series not only serves to minimize heat by physical separation but also allows treatment of significant lengths of calcification within the lesion such that therapy can be delivered expeditiously to minimize ischemic time.

Preclinical studies using micro-computed tomography

Experiments performed in cadaveric heavily calcified, excised human superficial femoral arteries identified unique mechanisms of IVL including modification of both superficial and deep calcium. Micro-computed tomography (CT) has demonstrated circumferential, transverse, and longitudinal calcium fractures with involvement of both superficial and deep layers of the vessel following IVL treatment.[17] Coregistration of micro-CT and histopathology identified multiple full-thickness and deep calcium fractures that did not traverse to the luminal surface. Magnified histopathology images revealed microfractures in both the superficial and deep layers of the artery. These findings support reports of improved stent expansion, even in the absence of visualized calcium fractures on intravascular imaging, suggesting that nontangential calcium fractures may also decrease calcium thickness and facilitate vascular compliance.

Clinical Studies: Results of CAD I to IV Optical Coherent Tomography Analysis

The Disrupt coronary artery disease (CAD) I, II, and III and Disrupt PAD II OCT substudies demonstrated calcium fracture following IVL treatment in vivo.[16,21,30] These OCT substudies uniformly demonstrated that the mechanism of lumen gain following IVL treatment is calcium fracture (both circumferential and longitudinal) with subsequent augmentation in vascular compliance and fracture expansion[17] following stent implantation. These observations suggest that calcium fracture is the likely mechanism by which IVL enhances vessel compliance and facilitates optimal stent expansion. A tercile analysis stratified by calcium burden in the Disrupt CAD I OCT substudy demonstrated similar stent expansion (>100%) at the site of maximum calcium thickness, regardless of the calcium angle.[21] Calcium fracture was observed in 67.7% of lesions after IVL in Disrupt CAD III.

Coronary Intravascular Lithotripsy Clinical Trials

Coronary IVL as adjunct to drug-eluting stent (DES) implantation in de novo calcified coronary stenosis was evaluated in the 4 Disrupt CAD clinical trials.[16,18–20] Study designs, subject inclusion/exclusion criteria, and outcomes of these studies have previously been described.[16,18–20,30] All Disrupt CAD studies were prospective, multicenter, and single-arm with the objective to evaluate the safety and effectiveness of coronary IVL before stent implantation for stable or unstable angina or silent ischemia due to severely calcified de novo coronary lesions. The major features of each study are shown in Table 1. The definition of severe calcification required the presence of fluoroscopic radiopacities without cardiac motion, before contrast injection, involving both sides of the arterial wall with a total length of calcium greater than or equal to 15 mm extending partially into the target lesion or intervascular imaging demonstration of a calcium angle greater than or equal to 270° in at least one cross section. Post-PCI, dual antiplatelet therapy was prescribed for a minimum of 6 months. Complete 30-day and 1-year follow-up is available for all studies. The pivotal trial for US regulatory approval, Disrupt CAD III, had a primary safety end point of freedom from major adverse cardiac events (MACE; composite occurrence of cardiac death, MI, or target vessel revascularization) at 30 days following PCI and a primary effectiveness end point of procedural success defined as successful stent delivery in a residual stenosis (% RS) less than 50% by core laboratory assessment without in-hospital MACE. A sensitivity analysis included procedural success with a % RS less than or equal to 30%. The Disrupt CAD III primary safety and effectiveness end points were based on the ORBIT II single-arm pivotal trial for orbital atherectomy regulatory approval that enrolled a similar patient population, had similar primary end points and definitions, and used a performance goal design. The ORBIT II primary safety and effectiveness results were used as the expected rates for CAD III to maintain a feasible sample size and to allow for a risk ratio of 1.5 consistent with US Food and Drug Administration guidance in other contemporary device studies. Disrupt CAD III enrolled 431 total patients (47 "roll-in" patients and 384 intention-to-treat [ITT]) at 47 international sites. In the ITT population, the average target lesion length was 26.1 ± 11.7 mm, total calcified segment length was 47.9 ± 18.8 mm, and all lesions were core laboratory adjudicated to be severely calcified. From the subset of patients (n = 100) enrolled into the OCT imaging substudy, the average calcium angle was 293 ± 77° and maximum calcium thickness was 0.96 ± 0.25 mm. The primary safety and effectiveness end points were achieved in 92.2% and 92.4% of the ITT population,

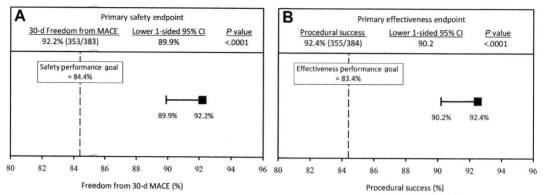

Fig. 2. Primary safety and effectiveness end points compared with their performance goals. (*A*) The primary safety end point was freedom from 30-day MACE, defined as cardiac death, myocardial infarction, or target vessel revascularization. The rate of the primary safety end point was 92.2% with a 1-sided lower 95% confidence interval of 89.9%, which was greater than the predefined performance goal of 84.4% ($P < .0001$). (*B*) The primary effectiveness end point was procedural success, defined as successful stent delivery with a residual stenosis less than 50% by angiographic core laboratory analysis without in-hospital MACE. The rate of the primary effectiveness end point was 92.4% with a one-sided lower 95% confidence interval of 90.2%, which was greater than the predefined performance goal of 83.4% ($P < .0001$). Thus, both the primary safety and effectiveness end points were met. CI, confidence interval. (*Reprinted from* Hill JM, Kereiakes DJ, Shlofmitz RA, et al. Intravascular lithotripsy for treatment of severely calcified coronary artery disease. J Am Coll Cardiol 2020;76(22):2635–46.)

respectively, and significantly exceeded the pre-specified performance goals of 84.4% and 83.4%, respectively (Fig. 2). Procedural success using a %RS threshold of less than or equal to 30% was observed in 92.2% of patients. Despite the severity of target lesion calcification, postprocedural in-stent %RS was less than or equal to 30% in 99.5% of lesions and serious angiographic complications were observed in only 2 patients (0.5%) at the end of the procedure. Specifically, perforation, abrupt vessel closure, and no reflow were not observed following IVL target lesion preparation alone. In the OCT substudy, the average stent expansion at the site of maximum lesion calcification was 102% ± 29% and the average MSA was 6.5 ± 2.1 mm². These remarkably salutary effects of IVL for target lesion preparation before DES implantation observed in CAD III were confirmed and extended in a patient-level pooled analysis involving the 628 patients enrolled into the CAD I to IV trials.[31] In this pooled patient cohort, the average target lesion length was 24.4 ± 11.5 mm, calcified segment length was 41.5 ± 20.0 mm, and 97% of all patients had core laboratory-adjudicated severe coronary calcification. Despite the severity of calcification, in-hospital and 30-day MACE rates were 6.5% and 7.3%, respectively, driven largely by the occurrence by periprocedural MI (defined by 3× upper limit normal (ULN) elevation of creatine kinase myocardial band isoenzyme (CK-MB)). Following IVL alone, perforation, abrupt closure, and no reflow were not observed (Fig. 3). Following subsequent

DES implantation, 0.2% of patients had a residual flow limiting dissection, minor perforation (Ellis classification I), or abrupt closure. Multivariable analysis identified clinical (history of MI) and target lesion-specific (lesion length ≥25 mm, bifurcation lesion) variables to be significant independent predictors of MACE and lack of procedural success for the pooled patient cohort. These excellent clinical and angiographic outcomes were remarkably consistent across all 4 trials involving 72 clinical sites in 12 countries. The benefit of IVL for target lesion preparation and to facilitate stent expansion is evident in the CAD I to IV pooled, patient-level OCT substudy analysis.[31] In this analysis of 262 patients, at the site of maximum target lesion calcification (as defined by arc), the average calcium arc was 270 ± 81° and thickness was 0.96 ± 0.25 mm.[32] Calcium fractures were visualized in 68% of cases (multiple in 48%), and the average stent expansion was 103% ± 29% with a MSA of 6.0 ± 1.9 mm².[33] Based on these measures of stent area and expansion, excellent longer-term outcomes might be predicted. Indeed, 1-year follow-up of Disrupt CAD III revealed a target lesion failure rate of 11.9% driven largely by periprocedural non-Q wave MI and low rates of target lesion revascularization (4.3%) and stent thrombosis (1.1%) to 1 year inclusive.[34]

Intravascular Lithotripsy-Induced Ventricular Capture

In the Disrupt CAD III trial, IVL-induced ventricular capture was commonly observed (41% of all cases)

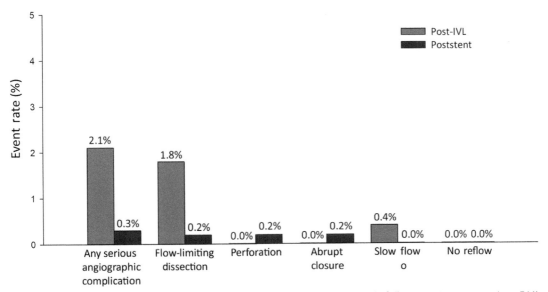

Fig. 3. Procedural angiographic outcomes following IVL treatment immediately following IVL treatment (n = 561) and post-stent (n = 628) demonstrated low rates of flow-limiting dissections (≥ grade D) with no perforation, abrupt closure, or no-reflow events following IVL treatment. (*Reprinted from Kereiakes DJ, Di Mario C, Riley RF, et al. Intravascular lithotripsy for treatment of calcified coronary lesions: patient-level pooled analysis of the Disrupt CAD studies. JACC Cardiovasc Interv 2021;14(12):1337–48.*)

but was without sustained arrhythmia or clinical sequalae. Multivariable Cox regression identified heart rate less than or equal to 60 beats/min, male sex, and total number of IVL pulses delivered as independent predictors of IVL-induced ventricular capture. IVL-induced capture results from mechanoelectric coupling of acoustic pressure waves with the cardiac conduction system that is mediated by cardiac stretch-activated channels used for conduction. Sustained ventricular capture is possible when the acoustic pressure waves depolarize the cardiac tissue via the stretch-activated response and the native heart rate is less than 60 beats/min or R-R intervals vary greater than 1 second. The resultant IVL-induced capture rate is 60 beats/min for the duration of IVL treatment (10 seconds). The probability of ventricular tachycardia (VT) or ventricular defibrillation (VF) induction by IVL is remote considering that the 8 µJ mechanical energy applied is several orders of magnitude lower than that used in standard implantable cardiac defibrillator (ICD) testing. In comparison, the electric energy required for VT or VF induction during testing of a newly implanted ICD is 0.6 to 2.0 J. Nevertheless, a single case report suggests the potential association of coronary IVL with VF induction but is confounded by the concurrent effects of balloon inflation-induced myocardial ischemia, spontaneous (not IVL related) ventricular ectopic effect on electric "vulnerability," and the use of IVL for an off-label

indication. As VF is a known risk in both coronary diagnostic and interventional procedures, especially in the presence of underlying myocardial ischemia, electrocardiographic monitoring is required during all coronary interventional procedures.

Intravascular Lithotripsy Learning Curve
Although every novel interventional technology has an operator learning curve, IVL leverages the familiarity of angioplasty balloon catheters used for coronary and peripheral intervention to provide an intuitively understandable and operator friendly procedure when treating complex calcified lesions. In Disrupt CAD III, the primary safety (freedom from MACE), primary effectiveness (procedural success without in-hospital MACE) end points, and device-lesion crossing success were not significantly different when comparing the first procedure from 47 international clinical sites (n = 47) with the subsequent 384 ITT procedures despite the complexity of lesions treated (Fig. 4). This observation underscores the relative ease of IVL use and general familiarity with the IVL delivery system (balloon catheter).

Intravascular Lithotripsy in Clinical Practice
The pooled individual patient data analysis from 4 Disrupt CAD studies demonstrated that IVL before DES implantation was associated with

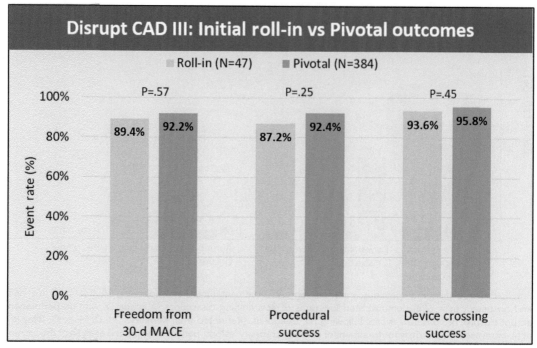

Fig. 4. Ease of IVL use. IVL device ease of use was demonstrated in Disrupt CAD III, because safety and effectiveness outcomes were similar between the initial IVL procedure (roll-in) at each participating site and subsequent IVL procedures (pivotal). (*Reprinted from* Kereiakes DJ, Virmani R, Hokama JY, et al. Principles of intravascular lithotripsy for calcific plaque modification. JACC Cardiovasc Interv 2021;14(12):1275–92.)

relatively low rates of in-hospital and 30-day MACE as well as high rates of procedural success that were similar across trials, geographies, and clinical sites with consistency of treatment effect across subgroups of patients (Fig. 5). In this regard, the treatment effect benefit of IVL, relative to atheroablation, was evident regardless of age, presence of diabetes mellitus, or chronic kidney disease.[34–37] Furthermore, this cumulative coronary experience with IVL confirmed the previously established relationship between target lesion length, bifurcation target lesions, and history of prior MI with both increased rates of MACE as well as reduced rates of procedural success. These readily available clinical and angiographic variables have demonstrated prognostic importance for safety and effectiveness of PCI and stent implantation with or without adjunctive atheroablation.[37,38] However, the safety and effectiveness of coronary IVL as demonstrated in clinical trials may not be generalizable to an "all comers," real-world practice. Indeed, specific clinical (acute coronary syndromes) and angiographic target lesion subsets (ostial, left main, nondilatable lesions, bypass grafts, in-stent restenosis, lesion length >40 mm, and so on) were not included in the CAD I to IV clinical trials. As the most

powerful predictor of in-stent restenosis is stent underexpansion, which is most often related to vessel calcification, IVL has been increasingly applied, without labeled indication, to achieve optimal stent expansion in this patient cohort.[39,4041] Furthermore, the combined use of IVL with atheroablative technologies was excluded from clinical trials and precludes understanding of the potential complementary utility of these technologies.[42] Data from ongoing "real-world" studies and the US postmarket study are required to address the limitations of clinical regulatory trials.

Expanded Use of Coronary Intravascular Lithotripsy

The role for coronary IVL is expanding beyond the previously limited inclusion criteria imposed by clinical trials. There are a multitude of ongoing studies evaluating IVL use in novel lesion subsets including in-stent restenosis, both left main and non-left main bifurcation lesions and IVL before DCB-only PCI. There are also prospective studies comparing the use of atherectomy (rotational and laser) versus cutting balloons versus IVL as stand-alone therapies for calcified coronary lesions as well as the safety of IVL use in sites without surgical backup. In

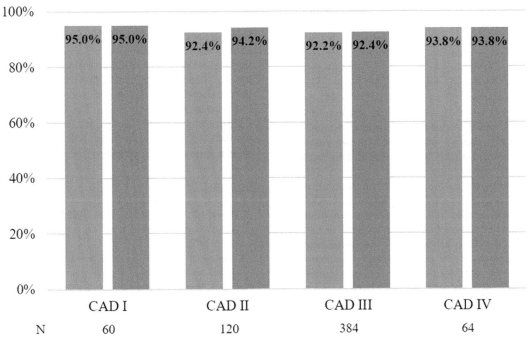

Fig. 5. Safety and effectiveness across the Disrupt CAD studies. Freedom from 30-day MACE is defined as freedom from the composite occurrence of cardiac death, myocardial infarction, or target vessel revascularization at 30 days. Procedural success is defined as successful stent delivery with a residual stenosis less than 50% by core laboratory assessment. (*Reprinted from* Kereiakes DJ, Virmani R, Hokama JY, et al. Principles of intravascular lithotripsy for calcific plaque modification. JACC Cardiovasc Interv 2021;14(12):1275–92.)

addition, IVL has been used to safely facilitate large-bore catheter access in patients with peripheral arterial disease, including MCS use in higher-risk PCI and transcatheter aortic valve replacement (TAVR).[43,44,45]

"Real-World" and Postmarket Trials of Coronary Intravascular Lithotripsy

There are a variety of upcoming prospective postmarket studies evaluating use of IVL, including registry-based studies from the Netherlands, Italy, France, India, and Spain. In addition, there is a prospective, multicenter, observational single-arm postapproval registry study in the United States that will use the National Cardiovascular Data Registry (NCDR) Cath PCI Registry. This NCDR study will use specific added data fields to evaluate 1000 patients with clinical characteristics similar to those enrolled into the Disrupt CAD III investigational device exemption trial. Technical success and safety end points will be evaluated to 30 days,

including a planned analysis of any IVL-related arrhythmias as well as the safety of IVL use in patients with permanent pacemakers and ICDs. Given the consistency of the pooled analysis of the Disrupt CAD I to IV studies, the hope is that these "real-world" studies will confirm the excellent safety and effectiveness profile for IVL use in calcified coronary lesions.[45]

SUMMARY

By building upon the principles of ESWL used for kidney stone fragmentation, the IVL acoustic waveform has been modified for safe and effective use in the treatment of vascular calcification. Evidence from both preclinical and clinical studies consistently supports the concept that IVL modifies both superficial and deep calcium by producing multiplane, circumferential, and longitudinal calcium fractures with consequent fracture expansion, increasing transmural vessel compliance, following DES implantation. The cumulative experience from clinical trials of coronary IVL target lesion preparation before DES implantation has demonstrated the relative safety of IVL compared with other methods used for coronary calcium modification with very low rates of angiographic and/or clinical adverse outcomes. Furthermore, coronary IVL effectiveness is reflected by the high rates of procedural success in conjunction with intravascular imaging measures of optimized DES deployment (% stent expansion, MSA) despite the presence of severe target lesion and vessel calcification. Indeed, perforation, abrupt vessel closure, and no-reflow have not been observed following target lesion preparation with IVL alone. Finally, late clinical outcomes seem to be excellent following IVL target lesion preparation and optimized DES implantation. Ongoing clinical studies will demonstrate the generalizability of clinical trial results to "real-world" clinical practice as well as the application of coronary IVL to patient (acute coronary syndromes) and target lesion cohorts (ostial, left main, nondilatable lesions, bypass grafts, in-stent restenosis, lesion lengths >40 mm, and so on) not included in clinical trials. In addition, because combined use of atheroablative technologies with IVL was excluded from the Disrupt CAD clinical trials, further investigation is required to understand the potential complementary utility of these technologies. Last, very late (beyond 1-year) clinical outcomes following coronary IVL as well as the application of IVL to severely calcified upper extremity vessels (ie, carotid, subclavian/axillary, innominate, radial and brachial) requires further study.

CLINICS CARE POINTS

- Severe coronary lesion calcification impedes stent delivery and optimal stent implantation leading to stent malapposition and underexpansion, which is associated with worse clinical outcomes including stent thrombosis and restenosis.

- IVL modifies vascular calcium with acoustic shockwaves that produce circumferential and longitudinal calcium fractures, which facilitates stent implantation.

- Coronary IVL before stent implantation is associated with low rates of clinical and angiographic complications and favorable measures of stent expansion/MSA by intravascular imaging.

DISCLOSURE STATEMENT

Dean Kereiakes states he is a consultant for Shockwave Medical, Elixir Medical, Svelte Medical, and Orchestra Biomed, Inc. Ziad Ali states he receives support from NIH/NHLBI, Abbott Vascular and Cardiovascular Systems Inc; personal fees from Amgen, Astra Zeneca, and Boston Scientific; and equity from Shockwave Medical. Robert Riley states he is a member of the speakers' bureau and is a consultant for Shockwave Medical, Inc and Boston Scientific Corporation. Timothy Smith states he has no conflicts to disclose. Richard Shlofmitz states he is a speaker for Shockwave Medical, Inc.

REFERENCES

1. Chen NX, Moe SM. Vascular calcification: pathophysiology and risk factors. Curr Hypertens Rep 2012;14(3):228–37.

2. Madhavan MV, Tarigopula M, Mintz GS, et al. Coronary artery calcification: pathogenesis and prognostic implications. J Am Coll Cardiol 2014;63(17):1703–14.

3. Wiemer M, Butz T, Schmidt W, et al. Scanning electron microscopic analysis of different drug eluting stents after failed implantation: from nearly undamaged to major damaged polymers. Catheter Cardiovasc Interv 2010;75(6):905–11.

4. Tzafriri AR, Garcia-Polite F, Zani B, et al. Calcified plaque modification alters local drug delivery in the treatment of peripheral atherosclerosis. J Control Release 2017;264:203–10.

5. Kobayashi Y, Okura H, Kume T, et al. Impact of target lesion coronary calcification on stent expansion. Circ J 2014;78(9):2209–14.

6. Mintz GS. Intravascular imaging of coronary calcification and its clinical implications. JACC Cardiovasc Imaging 2015;8(4):461–71.

7. Généreux P, Madhaven MV, Mintz GS, et al. Ischemic outcomes after coronary intervention of calcified vessels in acute coronary syndromes. Pooled analysis from the HORIZONS-AMI (Harmonizing Outcomes With Revascularization and Stents in Acute Myocardial Infarction) and ACUITY (Acute Catheterization and Urgent Intervention Triage Strategy) trials. J Am Coll Cardiol 2014;63(18):1845–54.

8. Chambers JW, Feldman RL, Himmelstein SI, et al. Pivotal trial to evaluate the safety and efficacy of the orbital atherectomy system in treating de novo, severely calcified coronary lesions (ORBIT II). JACC Cardiovasc Interv 2014;7(5):510–8.

9. Abdel-Wahab M, Toelg R, Byrne RA, et al. High-speed rotational atherectomy versus modified balloons prior to drug-eluting stent implantation in

severely calcified coronary lesions. Circ Cardiovasc Interv 2018;11(10):e007415.

10. Bourantas CV, Zhang YJ, Garg S, et al. Prognostic implications of coronary calcification in patients with obstructive coronary artery disease treated by percutaneous coronary intervention: a patient-level pooled analysis of 7 contemporary stent trials. Heart 2014;100(15):1158–64.

11. Sharma SK, Bolduan RW, Patel MR, et al. Impact of calcification on percutaneous coronary intervention: MACE-trial 1-year results. Catheter Cardiovasc Interv 2019;94(2):187–94.

12. Konigstein M, Madhaven MV, Ben-Yehuda O, et al. Incidence and predictors of target lesion failure in patients undergoing contemporary DES implantation-Individual patient data pooled analysis from 6 randomized controlled trials. Am Heart J 2019;213:105–11.

13. Guedeney P, Claessen BE, Mehran R, et al. Coronary calcification and long-term outcomes according to drug-eluting stent generation. J Am Coll Cardiol 2020;13(12):1417–28.

14. Kini AS, Vengrenyuk Y, Pena J, et al. Optical coherence tomography assessment of the mechanistic effects of rotational and orbital atherectomy in severely calcified coronary lesions. Catheter Cardiovasc Interv 2015;86(6):1024–32.

15. Yamamoto MH, Maehara A, Karimi Galougahi K, et al. Mechanisms of orbital versus rotational atherectomy plaque modification in severely calcified lesions assess by optical coherence tomography. J Am Coll Cardiol 2017;10(24):2584–6.

16. Ali ZA, Nef H, Escaned J, et al. Safety and effectiveness of coronary intravascular lithotripsy for treatment of severely calcified coronary stenoses: The Disrupt CAD II Study. Circ Cardiovasc Interv 2019; 12(10):e008434.

17. Kereiakes DJ, Virmani R, Hokama JY, et al. Principles of intravascular lithotripsy for calcific plaque modification. JACC Cardiovasc Interv 2021;14(12): 1275–92.

18. Brinton TJ, Ali ZA, Hill JM, et al. Feasibility of Shockwave coronary intravascular lithotripsy for the treatment of calcified coronary stenoses: first description. Circulation 2019;139(6):834–6.

19. Hill JM, Kereiakes DJ, Shlofmitz RA, et al. Intravascular lithotripsy for treatment of severely calcified coronary artery disease. J Am Coll Cardiol 2020; 76(22):2635–46.

20. Saito S, Yamazaki S, Takahashi A, et al. Intravascular lithotripsy for vessel preparation in severely calcified coronary arteries prior to stent placement: primary outcomes from the Japanese Disrupt CAD IV study. Circ J 2021;85(6):826–33.

21. Ali ZA, Brinton TJ, Hill JM, et al. Optical coherence tomography characterization of coronary lithotripsy

for treatment of calcified lesions: first description. JACC Cardiovasc Imaging 2017;10(8):897–906.

22. Blachutzik F, Honton B, Escaned J, et al. Safety and effectiveness of coronary intravascular lithotripsy in eccentric calcified lesions: a patient-level pooled analysis from the Disrupt CAD I and CAD II studies. Clin Res Cardiol 2021;110(2):228–36.

23. Wang Y, Osborne MT, Tung B, et al. Imaging cardiovascular calcification. J Am Heart Assoc 2018; 9(13):e008564.

24. Mori H, Torii S, Kutyna M, et al. Coronary artery calcification and its progression: what does it really mean? JACC Cardiovasc Imaging 2018;11(1):127–42.

25. Fujino A, Mintz GS, Matsumura M, et al. A new optical coherence tomography-based calcium scoring system to predict stent underexpansion. EuroIntervention 2018;13(18):e2182–9.

26. Riley RF, Henry TD, Mahmud E, et al. SCAI position statement on optimal percutaneous coronary interventional therapy for complex coronary artery disease. Catheter Cardiovasc Interv 2020;96(2):346–62.

27. Cleveland RO, McAteer JA. Physics of shock-wave lithotripsy. In: Smith AD, Badlani GH, Preminger GM, et al, editors. Smith's textbook of endourology. NJ: Wiley-BlackwellHoboken; 2012. p. 527–58.

28. Galougahi KK, Patel S, Shlofmitz RA, et al. Calcific plaque modification by acoustic shock waves: Intravascular lithotripsy in coronary interventions. Circ Cardiovasc Interv 2021;14(1):e009354.

29. Dini CS, Tomberli B, Mattesini A, et al. Intravascular lithotripsy for calcific coronary and peripheral artery stenoses. EuroIntervention 2019;15(8):714–21.

30. Kereiakes DJ, Hill JM, Ben-Yehuda O, et al. Evaluation of safety and efficacy of coronary intravascular lithotripsy for treatment of severely calcified coronary stenoses: Design and rationale for the Disrupt CAD III trial. Am Heart J 2020;225:10–8.

31. Kereiakes DJ, Di Mario C, Riley RF, et al. Intravascular lithotripsy for treatment of calcified coronary lesions: patient-level pooled analysis of the Disrupt CAD studies. JACC Cardiovasc Interv 2021;14(12):1337–48.

32. Ali Z, Hill J, Saito S, et al. Intravascular lithotripsy is effective in the treatment calcified nodules: patient-level pooled analysis from the disrupt CAD OCT sub-studies. J Am Coll Cardiol 2021; 78(19_Supplement_S):B51.

33. Ali ZA, Hill J, Saito S, et al. Optical coherence tomography characterization of eccentric versus concentric calcium treated with shockwave intravascular lithotripsy: patient-level pooled analysis of the disrupt CAD OCT sub-studies. J Am Coll Cardiol 2021;78(19_Supplement_S):B67–8.

34. Kereiakes DJ, Hill JM, Shlofmitz RA, et al, on behalf of the Disrupt CAD III Investigators. Kereiakes DJ on behalf of the Disrupt CAD III investigators. Intravascular Lithotripsy for Treatment of Severely Calcified

Coronary Lesions: 1-Year Results From the Disrupt CAD III Study. Journal of the Society for Cardiovascular Angiography & Intervention 2022;1(1). https://doi.org/10.1016/j.jscai.2021.100001.

35. Lee MS, Beasley R, Adams GL. Impact of advanced age on procedural and cute angiographic outcomes in patients treated for peripheral artery disease with orbital atherectomy: A CONFIRM registries subanalysis. J Invasive Cardiol 2015; 27(8):381–6.

36. Lee MS, Martinsen BJ, Lee AC, et al. Impact of diabetes mellitus on procedural and one year clinical outcomes following treatment of severely calcified coronary lesions with the orbital atherectomy system: A subanalysis of the ORBIT II study. Catheter Cardiovasc Interv 2018;91(6):1018–125.

37. Lee MS, Lee AC, Shlofmitz RA, et al. ORBIT II subanalysis: Impact of impaired renal function following treatment of severely calcified coronary lesions with the Orbital Atherectomy System. Catheter Cardiovasc Interv 2017;89(5):841–8.

38. Dangas GD, Serruys PW, Kereiakes DJ, et al. Meta-analysis of everolimus-eluting versus paclitaxel-eluting stents in coronary artery disease: final 3-year results of the SPIRIT clinical trials program (Clinical Evaluation of the Xience V Everolimus Eluting Coronary Stent System in the Treatment of Patients With De Novo Native Coronary Artery Lesions). JACC Cardiovasc Interv 2013; 6(9):914–22.

39. Kumar G, Shin EY, Sachdeva R, et al. Orbital atherectomy for the treatment of long ($\geq$25-40 mm) severely calcified coronary lesions: ORBIT II subanalysis. Cardiovasc Revasc Med 2020;21(2): 164–70.

40. Tizón-Marcos H, Rodríguez-Costoya I, Tevar C, et al. Intracoronary lithotripsy for calcific neoatherosclerotic in-stent restenosis: a case report. Eur Heart J Case Rep 2020;4(4):1–4.

41. Alfonso F, Bastante T, Antuña P, et al. Coronary lithotripsy for the treatment of undilatable calcified de novo and in-stent restenosis lesions. JACC Cardiovasc Interv 2019;12(5):497–9.

42. Chen G, Zrenner B, Pyxaras SA. Combined rotational atherectomy and intravascular lithotripsy for the treatment of severely calcified in-stent neoatherosclerosis: a mini-review. Cardiovasc Revasc Med 2019;20(9):819–21.

43. Nardi G, De Backer O, Saia F, et al. Peripheral intravascular lithotripsy of iliofemoral arteries to facilitate transfemoral TAVI: a multicentre prospective registry. EuroIntervention 2021;17. https://doi.org/10.4244/EIJ-D-21-00581.

44. Riley RF, Corl JD, Kereiakes DJ. Intravascular lithotripsy-assisted Impella insertion: A case report. Catheter Cardiovasc Interv 2019;93(7):1317–9.

45. Riley RF, Kolski B, Devireddy CM, et al. Percutaneous Impella Mechanical Circulatory Support Delivery Using Intravascular Lithotripsy. J Am Coll Cardiol Case Rep 2020;2(2):250–4.

Coronary Bifurcation Lesions

Zhen Ge, MD[1], Xiao-Fei Gao, MD[1], Jun-Jie Zhan, MD, PhD*, Shao-Liang Chen, MD*

KEYWORDS

- Coronary bifurcation lesions • Provisional stenting • Double kissing crush • Definition criteria

KEY POINTS

- Drug-eluting stent (DES) for coronary bifurcation lesions (CBLs) is commonly associated with suboptimal clinical results compared with nonbifurcation lesions.
- Provisional stenting (PS) is considered the preferred strategy for most of the CBLs.
- Double kissing (DK) crush is superior to PS in patients with complex left main (LM)-CBLs or non–LM-CBLs stratified by the DEFINITION criteria.

INTRODUCTION

Coronary bifurcation lesions (CBLs) are defined as coronary artery stenotic lesions involving the origin of significant side branches (SB).[1] Coronary bifurcated vessel segments are prone to develop atherosclerotic plaques due to turbulent blood flow and subsequent abnormal endothelial shear stress.[2] Among patients who undergo percutaneous coronary intervention (PCI), the prevalence of CBLs varies from 15% to 20%.[3] However, PCI using modern drug-eluting stents (DES) for the treatment of CBLs is still technically demanding, mainly due to the high rates of both acute and chronic complications compared with non-CBLs stenting.[4]

CLASSIFICATION OF CORONARY BIFURCATION LESIONS

The Medina classification is the most common classification of CBLs and offers a simple way to describe bifurcations.[5] CBLs consist of a proximal main vessel (MV), distal MV, and SB. The Medina classification assigns a binary score of 0 or 1 for the absence and presence of a stenosis in each segment of bifurcations in a clockwise sequence. A true CBL is defined as Medina class 1,1,1 and 1,0,1 or 0,1,1. Although the Medina classification is popular and easy to use, it does not provide some key information, such as plaque morphology, the extent of disease, the length of the MV and SB lesions, the presence or absence of thrombus, vessel diameter and angulation, which are relevant to decision making in the treatment of CBLs. Furthermore, a Medina 1,0,1 lesion is not accepted as a true bifurcation lesion, as it mirrors to Medina 1,1,0. On the other hand, several other classifications are not world widely studied.

CLASSIFICATION OF COMPLEX BIFURCATION LESIONS

Provisional stenting (PS) is a preferred strategy for most of the CBLs.[6] However, patients with complex CBLs undergoing PS may have an increased risk of SB occlusion or target lesion failure (TLF).[7] Decision-making in the treatment of CBLs should consider the complexity of CBLs. At present, several classifications have been introduced to guide the selection of an appropriate stenting technique and to predict the risk of SB compromise or clinical adverse events.

The RESOLVE risk score system consisting of 6 baseline angiographic variables independently predicts SB occlusion during PCI procedures, including TIMI flow of the MV, plaque distribution, diameter stenosis in the bifurcation core,

Nanjing First Hospital, Nanjing Medical University, No. 68 Changle Road, Nanjing 210006, Jiangsu, China
[1]Drs Z. Ge and X-F. Gao contributed equally to this work.
* Corresponding authors.
E-mail addresses: jameszll@163.com (J.-J.Z.); chmengx@126.com (S.-L.C.)

Intervent Cardiol Clin 11 (2022) 405–417
https://doi.org/10.1016/j.iccl.2022.02.002

bifurcation angle, the diameter ratio of MV to SB, and the extent of SB diameter stenosis.[8] The sum of the scores attributed to each variable can predict the risk of SB occlusion. Based on the RESOLVE score system, an SB protection strategy is recommended for CBLs with a high risk of SB occlusion, and a planned two-stent strategy is recommended for CBLs with larger caliber SB.

The 2018 ESC/EACTS guidelines on myocardial revascularization recommend an upfront two-stent approach for CBLs with[1]: an SB diameter ≥2.75 mm, and[2] SB lesion length greater than 5 mm, or[3] anticipated difficulty in accessing the SB after MV stenting, and[4] distal true left main (LM) bifurcation.[6,9] For distal LM bifurcation lesions, the DK crush technique is preferable to PS due to the potential risk of severe adverse events after SB occlusion.[6]

The DEFINITION criteria effectively differentiate simple from complex CBLs and help guide the treatment strategy for CBLs.[7,10] The DEFINITION criteria consist of 2 major and 6 minor angiographic criteria. Of the 2 major criteria, the requirement is SB lesion length ≥10 mm plus SB diameter stenosis ≥70% (for LM-CBLs) or SB diameter stenosis ≥90% (for non–LM-CBLs). Six minor criteria consist of moderate to severe calcification, multiple lesions, bifurcation angle less than 45° or greater than 70°, MV reference vessel diameter (RVD) < 2.5 mm, thrombus-containing lesions, and MV lesion length ≥25 mm. One major criterion plus any 2 minor criteria are required to define complex CBLs. A recent meta-analysis further reported that the SB lesion length ≥10 mm is a key predictor of stent failure after the PS approach.[11]

INTRACORONARY IMAGING GUIDANCE

Coronary angiography is often ambiguous for assessing lesion features at the ostium of the SB, lesion distribution, rewiring position, and stent expansion. Intravascular ultrasound (IVUS) and optical coherence tomography (OCT) are the 2 most commonly used tools for guiding stent implantation and optimizing stent expansion. A previous study has shown that intravascular imaging-guided PCI may improve clinical outcomes for complex CBLs.[12] The ULTIMATE study demonstrated that IVUS-guided PCI reduced the risk of target vessel failure (TVF) compared with angiography-guided PCI at the 1-year follow-up.[13] The subgroup analysis also showed that IVUS guidance had a trend toward greater clinical benefits than angiography guidance for patients with CBLs. In that study, 3

IVUS-derived optimal criteria were prespecified[1]: expansion index greater than 0.9, or minimal stent area (MSA) in the stented segment is > 5.0 mm[22]; plaque burden 5-mm proximal or distal to the stent edge is less than 50%; and[3] no edge dissection involving media with a length greater than 3 mm. However, the optimization criteria for IVUS-guided PCI for CBLs are currently inconclusive. For LM-CBLs, Kang and colleagues[14] reported that the cut-off of MSA measured by IVUS was 5-6-7-8 mm^2 at the ostium of the LCX-LAD-POC-LM shaft, respectively, independently predicting the clinical events. However, the EXCEL study showed that the IVUS-derived optimal MSA was 6-7-10 mm^2 at the LCX-LAD-LM, respectively.[15] Additionally, the IVUS-derived optimal criteria for non–LM-CBLs remain understudied. The DKCRUSH-VIII trial (NCT03770650) is to determine the superiority of IVUS-guided versus angiography-guided DK crush stenting for patients with complex CBLs according to the DEFINITION criteria.[16] The prespecified optimal criteria of IVUS-guided PCI for LM-CBLs or non–LM-CBLs determined in the DKCRUSH-VIII trial will provide solid data on how to further optimize DK crush stenting for CBLs. The OCTOBER trial (NCT03171311) is a prospective, multicenter, randomized controlled study, which aims to compare the superiority of OCT-guided PCI with angiography-guided PCI in patients with true CBLs treated with either PS or a planned two-stent technique.[17] Given a pool of data from observational studies, randomized clinical trials(RCTs) will further enhance the importance of intravascular imaging-guided bifurcation stenting.

PHYSIOLOGIC EVALUATION
Fractional Flow Reserve
Fractional flow reserve (FFR) refers to the ratio of distal coronary artery pressure (Pd) to the aortic pressure (Pa) in the state of hyperemia. FFR is the gold standard for evaluating the functional significance of coronary artery disease.[6,18] FFR-guided jailed SB interventional strategy for CBLs has been shown to result in good functional outcomes and less frequent SB interventions, with no significant difference in the short-term clinical outcomes compared with the conventional strategy.[19,20] However, due to the less favorable performance of the pressure wire and the complicated anatomic features of CBLs, the DKCRUSH VI study has reported that the failure rate of SB FFR measurement after stenting the MV was up to 9%.[20] LM-CBLs are often involved in the ostium of LAD or LCX

and are accompanied with more frequent downstream lesions. The severity of LM lesions is usually underestimated in the presence of downstream lesions.[21] To date, there is a lack of large-scale randomized controlled trials (RCTs) to validate the clinical application of FFR-guided interventional strategies for LM-CBLs.

Quantitative Flow Ratio

The application of FFR for the physiologic evaluation of SB is limited due to the challenge of SB FFR measurement after MV stenting,[20] the need for hyperemia and high cost, and the potential risk of pressure wire–induced complications. The quantitative flow ratio (QFR) is a novel tool for the physiologic assessment of coronary artery disease based on 2 angiographic views.[22] The diagnostic performance and prognostic value of the QFR have been previously validated.[23,24] Nevertheless, the diagnostic accuracy of the QFR in the assessment of CBLs is decreased by assuming a linear tapering of the reference vessel size.[22] The uQFR is a new method for computing the QFR based on Murray's fractal law from a single projection of angiography, and is empowered by artificial intelligence for automatic delineation of major coronary arteries and their SBs.[25] The feasibility and diagnostic accuracy of the μQFR have been tested recently,[25] but the clinical relevance of the SB QFR in patients with CBLs requires further study.

Stenting Approaches for Bifurcation Lesions

Multiple RCTs have assessed the clinical effects of PS versus planned two-stent techniques for CBLs.[26–31] Most of these studies have shown that upfront two-stent techniques are associated with a higher risk of major adverse cardiac events (MACE) than PS, which provides evidence-based data to update guidelines and expert recommendations preferring PS for most CBLs. However, the DEFINITION II, DKCRUSH-II, and DKCRUSH-V trials related to the DK crush technique have shown that the planned two-stent technique is superior to PS for the treatment of CBLs.[10,30,32] The key randomized trials comparing PS with systematic two-stent techniques are presented in Table 1.[10,26–34] Two key factors should be considered before decision-making for the treatment of CBLs. One such factor is the complexity of bifurcation lesions. The DEFINITION study has reported that the complexity of CBLs is associated with clinical outcomes.[7] In particular, the length of SB lesions is a key factor affecting the clinical results of different stenting techniques. The DEFIITION criteria were developed from the DEFIITION study and validated in the DEFINITION-II study.[7,10] Upfront two-stent techniques are superior to PS in the reduction of TLF for complex CBLs stratified by the DEFIITION criteria. The other factor is that different two-stent techniques may have a wider discrepancy in the clinical outcomes. The DK crush technique has shown excellent performance in lowering TLF for both non–LM-CBLs and LM-CBLs compared with classic crush or culotte stenting.[35,36] The key randomized trials comparing different systematic two-stent techniques are presented in Table 2.[35–38]

STENTING TECHNIQUES OF BIFURCATION LESIONS

Provisional Stenting Technique

PS is a step-wise stenting technique, which is used for most of the CBLs (~70%). The first stent is initially implanted in the MV across the SB, and a second stent may be used as a bail-out two-stent strategy in cases whereby the SB is severely compromised, with or without diminished blood flow or dissection after MV stenting.

A 6 French guiding catheter and radial approach are suitable for most patients. Using a jailed wire to actively protect the SB depends on the risk of SB occlusion after MV stenting, the SB diameter, and difficult SB access. The clinical outcomes of the jailed balloon technique lack of evidence-based data. Routine SB predilatation is not recommended but may be considered if SB access is difficult or if there is severe SB disease in the ostial/proximal segment.[39] The MV stent size is always adjusted according to the distal RVD of the MV. The length of the proximal MV stent should be sufficiently long to allow the performance of the proximal optimization technique (POT). After MV stenting, the POT is performed using a short noncompliant balloon with a 1:1 ratio diameter of the proximal MV. Routine kissing balloon inflation (KBI) is not recommended but should be considered if any of the following apply[1]: SB TIMI flow less than 3,[2] FFR less than 0.8, or[3] SB dissection $\geq$ type B.[40] Rewiring through a distal cell of the MV stent is optimal to cover the ostium of the SB after KBI. The Re-POT should be performed to restore circular geometry and reduce stent strut malapposition in the MV.[41] After MV stenting, a bail-out stent may be needed if any of the following apply[1]: SB TIMI flow less than 3,[2] FFR less than 0.8, or[3] SB dissection $\geq$ type B. Based on the rewiring position, different two-stent techniques may be used. When rewiring through

Table 1
Key randomized trials comparing provisional stenting (PS) with systematic two-stent techniques

Trials	N	2-Stent Technique	SB Length (mm)		SB DS (%)		Primary Endpoint	Results (PS vs 2-stent)
			PS	2-Stent	PS	2-Stent		
NORDIC I	413	Classic crush, T, culotte	6.0 ± 4.8	6.4 ± 4.7	46 ± 26	47 ± 26	MACE (CD, MI, TVR, ST) at 6 mo	2.9% vs 3.4%
BBK I	101	T	10.4 ± 4.1	9.9 ± 4.2	53.1 ± 23.5	54.4 ± 22.3	% DS of SB at 9 mo	23.0% vs 27.7%
CACTUS	350	Classic crush	5.7 ± 4.2	5.9 ± 4.7	61 ± 13	63 ± 12	In-segment restenosis at 6 mo	MV: 6.7% vs 4.6% SB: 14.7% vs 13.2%
BBC ONE	500	Crush, culotte	-	-	-	-	MACE (death, MI, TVF) at 9 mo	8% vs 15.2%
DKCRUSH II	370	DK Crush	14.9 ± 12.5	15.4 ± 11.3	63.4 ± 14.2	62.8 ± 14.7	MACE (CD, MI, TVR) at 12 mo	17.3% vs 10.3%
EBC TWO	200	Culotte	9.7 ± 7.1	10.8 ± 7.3	54.1 ± 15.6	54.8 ± 13.9	MACE (death, MI, TVR) at 12 mo	7.7% vs 10.3%
Nordic-Baltic IV	450	Culotte, minicrush, T	6.4 ± 4.1	7.7 ± 4.9	43 ± 18	49 ± 17	MACE (CD, non-PMI, TLR, dST) at 6 mo	5.5% vs 2.2%
DKCRUSH V	482	DK Crush	16.6 ± 11.9	16.2 ± 14.0	65.3 ± 8.3	65.8 ± 7.5	TLF (CD, TVMI, TLR) at 1 y	10.7% vs 5.0%
DEFINITION II	653	DK Crush (77%), Culotte	19.9 ± 9.3	20.7 ± 10.1	61.5 ± 15.3	62.3 ± 15.8	TLF (CD, TVMI, TLR) at 1 y	11.4% vs 6.1%
EBC MAIN	467	Culotte, DK-minicrush, T or TAP	5.8 ± 4.0	7.9 ± 5.7	51.9 ± 18.5	55.4 ± 15.7	Death, MI, and TLR at 12 mo	14.7% vs 17.7%

Abbreviations: CD, cardiac death; DK, double kissing; DS, diameter stenosis; dST, definite stent thrombosis; MACE, major adverse cardiac events; MI, myocardial infarction; PMI, peri-procedural myocardial infarction; PS, provisional stenting; SB, side branch; ST, stent thrombosis; TAP, T, and small protrusion; TLF, target lesion failure; TLR, target lesion revascularization; TVMI, target vessel myocardial infarction; TVR, target vessel revascularization.

Table 2
Key randomized trials comparing different systematic two-stent techniques

Trials	N	LM-CBLs (%)	Arm1	Arm2	Primary Endpoint	Results Arm1 vs Arm2
DKCRUSH I	311	15%	Classic crush	DK crush	MACE (CD, MI, TVR) at 8 mo	24.4% vs 11.4%
Nordic II	424	10%	Culotte	Classic crush	MACE (CD, MI, TVR or ST) at 6 mo	3.7% vs 4.3%
BBK II	300	17%	Culotte	TAP	% DS at 9-mo angiographic follow-up.	21% vs 27%
DKCRUSH III	419	100%	DK crush	Culotte	MACE (CD, MI and TVR) at 1 y	6.2% vs 16.3%

Abbreviations: CD, cardiac death; DK, double kissing; DS, diameter stenosis; LM-CBLs, left main distal coronary bifurcation lesions; MACE, major adverse cardiac events; MI, myocardial infarction; ST, stent thrombosis; TAP, T and small protrusion; TLR, target lesion revascularization; TVR, target vessel revascularization.

the distal cell of the MV stent, the PS-T technique may be considered. When rewiring through the proximal MV stent strut, T and small protrusion (TAP) or reverse culotte stenting technique may avoid missing the ostium of the SB.[42] Re-POT is mandatory after SB stenting and final KBI. The steps for PS-T are shown in **Fig. 1**.

Two- Stent Techniques
Traditional T stenting technique
Traditional T stenting is an approach of the two-stent strategy family, which is suitable for bifurcation angles of more than 70^0 and can be used in either LM-CBLs or non–LM-CBLs. The SB stent is precisely implanted at the ostium of the SB with or without an MV balloon to help with precise positioning. Rewiring through the distal cell of the MV stent is followed by MV stenting and the final KBI must be performed after dilating the MV and SB stent sequentially. The main challenge of the T-stenting technique is a geographic miss at the ostium of the SB, which is associated with an increased MACE rate in long-term follow-up.[43] TAP is a modified T-stenting technique, for which the proximal part of the SB stent protrudes in the MV to completely cover the SB ostium after MV stenting.[44] There are no significant benefits in using upfront T-stenting over PS.[43]

Culotte stenting technique and double kissing mini-culotte stenting technique
The culotte technique is one of the systematic two-stent strategies, which shares a similar sequence with PS-T and is best suitable for type "Y" bifurcations with a similar diameter between the SB and MV.[45] The steps for the culotte stenting are shown in **Fig. 2**. The first

stent is recommended to be implanted in a branch with a wider angle or critical disease. The culotte stenting technique completely covers the SB ostium; however, double-layer stent struts overlapping at the proximal MV increase the risk of stent thrombosis. After rewiring through the distal cell of the first stent, the second stent is deployed in the second branch, with the proximal segments of the 2 stents overlapping each other. The POT is necessary after the final KBI. Owing to the limitations of the traditional culotte technique, such as overlapping double-layer stent struts in the proximal MV, need for type "Y" bifurcations, and a similar diameter between two daughter vessels, the DK mini-culotte technique is a modified culotte in 2 aspects[1]: shorter protrusion of the first stent into the MV (usually 1–2 mm), and[2] the first KBI will be performed after rewiring the first stent.[46] The DK mini-culotte technique is superior to PS for true bifurcation lesions.[47]

Double kissing crush stenting technique
The DK crush technique has been described previously.[35] The detailed DK crush stenting process is summarized as follows[1]: SB stenting: a stent with a stent/artery ratio of 1.1:1 is positioned in the SB, protruding into the MV 2 to 3 mm after adequately preparing target bifurcation lesions; a noncompliant balloon with a balloon/artery ratio of 1:1 is advanced in the MV and the SB stent is deployed; the stent balloon and SB wire is removed after confirming no complications in the SB by angiography[2]; balloon crushing: the MV balloon is inflated to crush the SB stent[3]; first KBI: after rewiring the SB from the proximal stent cell by visual estimation, 2 noncompliant balloons in both the SB and the MV are inflated to perform the first KBI[4]; MV

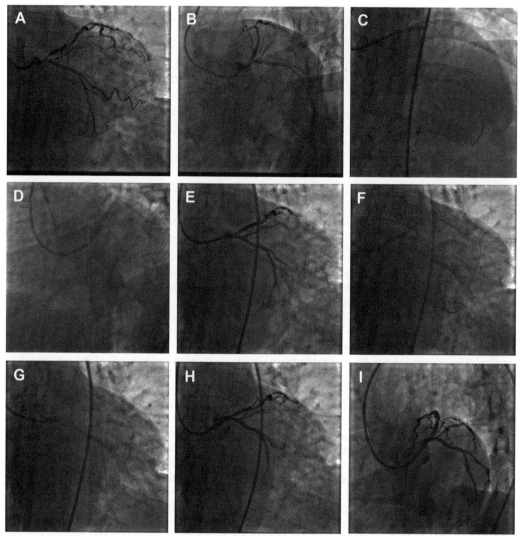

Fig. 1. A case using the provisional stenting technique. A 67-year-old man presented with unstable angina. (A, B) Angiography showing Medina 1,1,1 distal left main (LM) bifurcation lesions. (C) A 4.0 × 13 mm drug-eluting stent (DES) was deployed from the left anterior descending artery (LAD)-LM after predilating the LAD-LM. (D) The proximal optimization technique (POT) was performed with a 5.0 × 12 mm noncompliant (NC) balloon. (E, F) Kissing balloon inflation was performed with a 3.75 × 12 mm NC balloon in the LAD and a 3.5*12 mm NC balloon in the left circumflex artery (LCX) at 12 atm after rewiring the LCX from the distal stent cell. (G) re-POT with a 5.0 × 12 mm NC balloon. (H, I) Final results.

stenting: the second stent with a stent/artery ratio of 1.1:1 is deployed in the MV[5]; the first POT: a noncompliant balloon according to the proximal RVD is used to postdilate the proximal MV[6]; the final KBI: when rewiring the SB from the proximal stent cell, the final KBI has to be performed after postdilating the MV and the SB stent sequentially; and[7] re-POT: the steps for the DK crush stenting technique are shown in Fig. 3. The DK crush stenting technique involves balloon crushing, rewiring of the SB, double KBI, and POT; therefore, IVUS-guided DK

crush stenting may further optimize the PCI procedure and improve clinical outcomes. The detailed IVUS-guided DK crush stenting process is explained in detail in the DKCRUSH-VIII trial,[16] which is a prospective, RCT to compare IVUS-guided with angiography-guided DK crush stenting in patients with complex bifurcations stratified by the DEFINITION criteria.

Serial DKCRUSH trials have shown that DK crush significantly reduces the risk of revascularization, myocardial infarction (MI), or stent thrombosis for both non–LM-CBLs and LM-

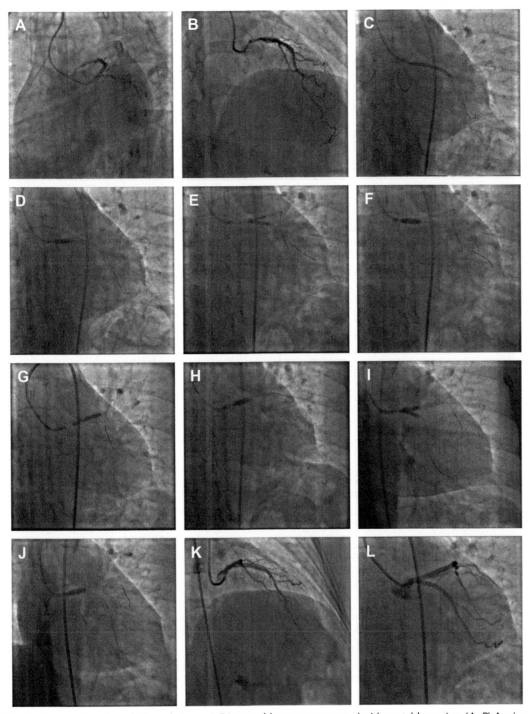

Fig. 2. A case using the culotte technique. A 54-year-old woman presented with unstable angina. (*A, B*) Angiography showing Medina 1,1,1 distal left main (LM) bifurcation lesions. (*C*) A 3.0 × 30 mm drug-eluting stent (DES) was inflated in the left circumflex artery (LCX)-LM through a 7-F guiding catheter. (*D*) A proximal optimization technique (POT) was performed with a 4.0 × 10 mm noncompliant (NC) balloon. (*E*) Kissing balloon inflation was performed with 2 NC balloons at 12 atm after rewiring the left anterior descending artery (LAD). (*F*) POT was performed with a 4.0 × 10 mm NC balloon. (*G*) A 3.5 × 24 mm DES was deployed from the LAD to the LM. (*H*) POT was performed with a 4.0 × 10 mm NC balloon. (*I*) Kissing balloon inflation was performed with a 3.0 × 12 mm NC balloon in the LCX and a 3.5*12 mm NC balloon in the LAD at 14 atm. (*J*) POT was performed with a 4.5 × 10 mm NC balloon. (*K, L*) Final results.

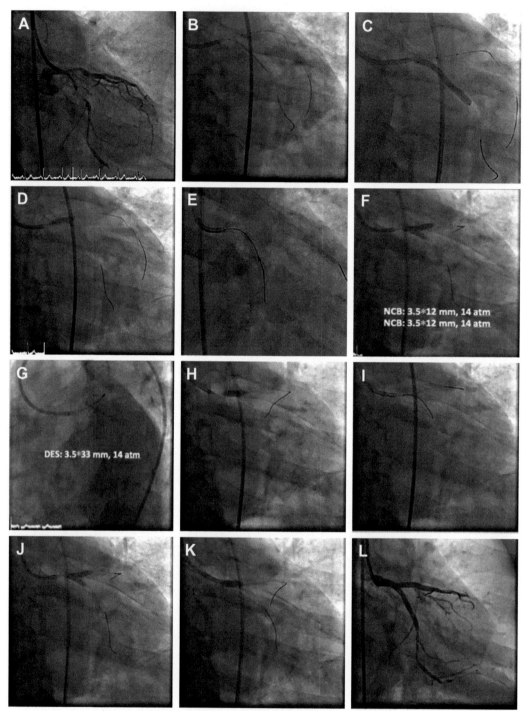

Fig. 3. A case using the double kissing (DK) crush technique. A 62-year-old man presented with unstable angina. (A) Angiography showing a Medina 1,1,1 distal left main (LM) bifurcation lesion. (B, C) A 3.5 × 29 mm drug-eluting stent (DES) was positioned in the left circumflex artery (LCX) with 2-mm protrusion into the LM. A 3.5 × 12 mm noncompliant (NC) balloon was embedded in the left anterior descending artery (LAD) through a 6-F guiding catheter before the LCX stent was deployed. (D) The NC balloon in the LAD was used to crush the LCX stent. (E, F) Kissing balloon inflation was performed with two 3.5 × 12 mm NC balloons at 14 atm after rewiring LCX. (G) A 3.5 × 33 mm DES was deployed from the LAD to the LM. (H) The proximal optimization technique (POT) was performed with a 4.0 × 12 mm NC balloon. (I, J) Final kissing balloon inflation was performed with two 3.5 × 12 mm NC balloons following NC balloon postdilating sequentially after rewiring the LCX. (K) Re-POT with a 4.0 × 12 mm NC balloon. (L) Final results.

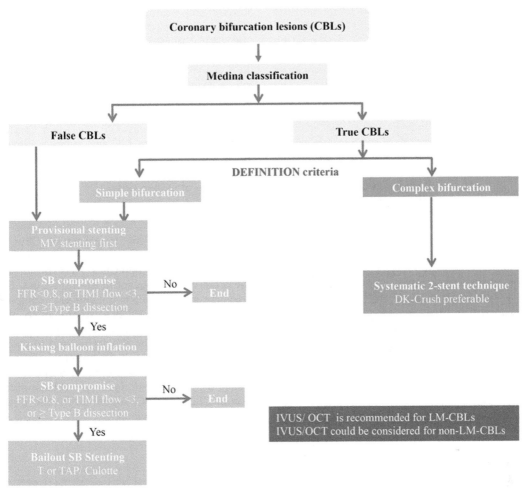

Fig. 4. Algorithm for coronary bifurcation lesions intervention. DK, double kissing, DS, diameter stenosis, IVUS, intravascular ultrasound, LM-CBLs, left main distal coronary bifurcation lesions, MV, main vessel, OCT, optical coherence tomography, RVD, reference vessel diameter, SB, side branch, TIMI, thrombolysis in myocardial infarction, T or TAP, T-stenting or T and small protrusion.

CBLs compared with PS, classic crush, or culotte.[10,32,35,36] The discrepancy in clinical outcomes between DKCURSH trials and previous RCTs reporting the superiority of PS over other two-stent techniques may be related to differences in the complexity of CBLs. As the DEFINITION II trial has reported, the systematic two-stent approach (DK crush: 77.8%) may improve clinical outcomes compared with PS in patients with complex bifurcation lesions according to the DEFINITION criteria.[10]

LEFT MAIN BIFURCATION LESIONS

Newer generation DES and techniques have improved clinical outcomes in patients with unprotected LM disease who undergo PCI. While PCI is recommended for the treatment of the distal true LM-CBLs, upfront two-stent strategies may be considered due to SB with a larger size and a wider angle. Subgroup analysis of the EXCEL trial demonstrated a higher rate of composite endpoint (death, MI, stroke) at 3 years in patients with LM-CBLs treated with the planned two-stent technique versus PS, driven by differences in cardiovascular death and MI.[48] Notably, in the subgroup analysis, no significant differences between the planned two-stent technique and PS were found in patients with distal true LM-CBLs. Furthermore, T or TAP and culotte stenting were the most commonly used two-stent techniques. The DKCRUSH-V trial demonstrated that the DK crush technique is superior to PS in the reduction of TLF in patients with unprotected LM-CBLs at 1- or 3-year follow-up.[32,49] The results of DKCRUSH-V support that DK crush may be suitable for LM-CBLs, as reflected by the current guideline recommendation that DK crush may be preferable for LM-CBLs.[6] However, the latest EBC MAIN trial has reported that PS is "non-inferior" to planned two-stent techniques in patients with unprotected LM-CBLs.[34] The EBC MAIN trial was initially designed as a superior study with overall neutral results; as a result, the conclusion of noninferiority is inconsistent with the original purpose of the principle investigator. Insight analysis from that trial, EBC MAIN also has some key drawbacks[1]: mean SB lesion length = 7 mm (inclusion requiring >8 mm)[2]; MI < 72 h or any chronic total occlusion (CTO) lesion not included[3]; mean SYNTAX score = 23[4]; 11% of difference in the assumption of 1-year primary endpoint between the 2 groups increased the bias and type II error[5]; myocardial biomarkers, an important element of the primary endpoint, was not measured in 15% of patients[6]; T, TAP and culotte stenting were the major two-stent techniques; and[7] operators were less experienced in LM-PCI. It seems that simpler LM-CBLs were studied in the EBC MAIN trial than in the DKCRUSH V study. Indeed, both the DKCRUSH-III and DKCRUSH-II trials have demonstrated that DK crush is superior to the culotte or PS-T/TAP technique in the reduction of MACE or TLF through a 3-year follow-up.[30,36,50,51] Further clinical benefits can be achieved by the application of the DK crush technique in complex LM-CBLs according to the DEFINITION criteria.[10,49]

DRUG-COATED BALLOON

Using a drug-coated balloon (DCB) to treat restenosis of CBLs, in particular, whereby they have been treated with the two-stent technique, has been extensively reported as an attractive approach that can improve the clinical outcomes and minimize multiple stent layers at the site of bifurcations.[52] The use of DCB in de novo CBLs includes the following[1]: using DCB to treat the MV and SB, implanting a bare metal stent into the MV[2]; using DCB to treat SB, implantation of a DES into the MV[3]; after MV DES implantation, treating SB with DCB; and[4] only using a DCB to treat the MV and SB. Current studies mainly focus on DES for the treatment of MV, and DCB for SB. The BEYOND study aimed to investigate the benefits of SB treatment with DCB compared with regular balloon angioplasty in patients with de novo non–LM-CBLs treated with PS, and showed that DCB was superior to a regular balloon in the reduction of lumen diameter stenosis and late lumen loss at the 9-month follow-up.[53] At present, data on DCB use in

CBLs mainly comes from surrogate endpoints, and there is a lack of large-scale RCTs to validate the clinical outcomes of DCB in CBLs. DCB-BIF(NCT04242134), a prospective, multicenter, RCT was designed to determine the superiority of DCB versus noncompliant balloon for the treatment of SB after PS in patients with simple CBLs stratified by the DEFINITION criteria. The primary endpoint was TVF (including cardiac death, target vessel MI, and clinically driven revascularization) at the 1-year follow-up. This study will provide solid data on the efficacy and safety of DCB in CBLs.

SUMMARY

PCI with DES for the treatment of CBLs is commonly associated with suboptimal clinical results compared with non-CBLs. PS is considered the preferred strategy for most of the CBLs. DK crush is superior to PS in patients with complex LM-CBLs or non–LM-CBLs according to the DEFINITION criteria. Intracoronary imaging and physiologic evaluation should be used to guide CBLs intervention to achieve better clinical outcomes. DCB may be a promising approach to treat CBLs, and further data support its application in CBLs. The PCI Algorithm for the treatment of CBLs is shown in **Fig. 4**.

CLINICS CARE POINTS

- PCI with DES for the treatment of CBLs is technically demanding, mainly because of higher rates of both acute and chronic complications as compared with non-CBLs stenting.
- PS is the default strategy for most CBLs.
- DK crush is associated with better clinical outcomes compared with PS in patients with complex LM-CBLs or non–LM-CBLs stratified by the DEFINITION criteria.
- Intracoronary imaging and/or physiologic evaluation are useful tools to guide the treatment of bifurcation lesions.
- Use of DCB in bifurcation lesions needs further data to support the clinical benefits.

ACKNOWLEDGMENTS

This work was funded by grants from the National Science Foundation of China [grant number NSFC 91639303 and NSFC 81770441] and jointly supported by Jiangsu Provincial Special Program of Medical Science (BE2019615). Dr. Shao-Liang Chen is a Fellow at the Collaborative Innovation Center for Cardiovascular Disease Translational Medicine, Nanjing Medical University, Nanjing, China.

DISCLOSURE

All authors report no relevant conflicts of interest

REFERENCES

1. Louvard Y, Thomas M, Dzavik V, et al. Classification of coronary artery bifurcation lesions and treatments: time for a consensus! Catheterization Cardiovasc interventions 2008;71:175–83.

2. Giannoglou G, Antoniadis A, Koskinas K, et al. Flow and atherosclerosis in coronary bifurcations. EuroIntervention 2010;J16–23.

3. Serruys P, Onuma Y, Garg S, et al. 5-year clinical outcomes of the ARTS II (Arterial Revascularization Therapies Study II) of the sirolimus-eluting stent in the treatment of patients with multivessel de novo coronary artery lesions. J Am Coll Cardiol 2010;55:1093–101.

4. Garot P, Lefevre T, Savage M, et al. Nine-month outcome of patients treated by percutaneous coronary interventions for bifurcation lesions in the recent era: a report from the Prevention of Restenosis with Tranilast and its Outcomes (PRESTO) trial. J Am Coll Cardiol 2005;46:606–12.

5. Medina A, Suárez de Lezo J, Pan M. [A new classification of coronary bifurcation lesions]. Revista espanola de cardiologia 2006;59:183.

6. Neumann FJ, Sousa-Uva M, Ahlsson A, et al. 2018 ESC/EACTS Guidelines on myocardial revascularization. Eur Heart J 2019;40:87–165.

7. Chen SL, Sheiban I, Xu B, et al. Impact of the complexity of bifurcation lesions treated with drug-eluting stents: the DEFINITION study (Definitions and impact of complEx biFurcation lesIons on clinical outcomes after percutaNeous coronary IntervenTIOn using drug-eluting steNts). JACC Cardiovasc Interv 2014;7:1266–76.

8. Dou K, Zhang D, Xu B, et al. An angiographic tool for risk prediction of side branch occlusion in coronary bifurcation intervention: the RESOLVE score system (Risk prEdiction of Side branch OccLusion in coronary bifurcation interVEntion). JACC Cardiovasc Interv 2015;8:39–46.

9. Lassen JF, Burzotta F, Banning AP, et al. Percutaneous coronary intervention for the left main stem and other bifurcation lesions: 12th consensus document from the European Bifurcation Club. EuroIntervention 2018;13:1540–53.

10. Zhang JJ, Ye F, Xu K, et al. Multicentre, randomized comparison of two-stent and provisional stenting techniques in patients with complex coronary bifurcation lesions: the DEFINITION II trial. Eur Heart J 2020;41:2523–36.

11. Di Gioia G, Sonck J, Ferenc M, et al. Clinical Outcomes Following Coronary Bifurcation PCI Techniques: A Systematic Review and Network Meta-Analysis Comprising 5,711 Patients. JACC Cardiovasc Interv 2020;13:1432–44.

12. Chen L, Xu T, Xue XJ, et al. Intravascular ultrasound-guided drug-eluting stent implantation is associated with improved clinical outcomes in patients with unstable angina and complex coronary artery true bifurcation lesions. Int J Cardiovasc Imaging 2018;34:1685–96.

13. Zhang J, Gao X, Kan J, et al. Intravascular Ultrasound Versus Angiography-Guided Drug-Eluting Stent Implantation: The ULTIMATE Trial. J Am Coll Cardiol 2018;72:3126–37.

14. Kang SJ, Ahn JM, Song H, et al. Comprehensive intravascular ultrasound assessment of stent area and its impact on restenosis and adverse cardiac events in 403 patients with unprotected left main disease. Circ Cardiovasc interventions 2011;4: 562–9.

15. Lee SY, Ahn JM, Mintz GS, et al. Ten-Year Clinical Outcomes of Late-Acquired Stent Malapposition After Coronary Stent Implantation. Arterioscler Thromb Vasc Biol 2020;40:288–95.

16. Ge Z, Kan J, Gao XF, et al. Comparison of intravascular ultrasound-guided with angiography-guided double kissing crush stenting for patients with complex coronary bifurcation lesions: Rationale and design of a prospective, randomized, and multicenter DKCRUSH VIII trial. Am Heart J 2021;234:101–10.

17. Holm NR, Andreasen LN, Walsh S, et al. Rational and design of the European randomized Optical Coherence Tomography Optimized Bifurcation Event Reduction Trial (OCTOBER). Am Heart J 2018;205:97–109.

18. De Bruyne B, Pijls N, Kalesan B, et al. Fractional flow reserve-guided PCI versus medical therapy in stable coronary disease. New Engl J Med 2012; 367:991–1001.

19. Koo B, Park K, Kang H, et al. Physiological evaluation of the provisional side-branch intervention strategy for bifurcation lesions using fractional flow reserve. Eur Heart J 2008;29:726–32.

20. Chen SL, Ye F, Zhang JJ, et al. Randomized Comparison of FFR-Guided and Angiography-Guided Provisional Stenting of True Coronary Bifurcation Lesions: The DKCRUSH-VI Trial (Double Kissing Crush Versus Provisional Stenting Technique for Treatment of Coronary Bifurcation Lesions VI). JACC Cardiovasc Interv 2015;8:536–46.

21. Fearon WF, Yong AS, Lenders G, et al. The impact of downstream coronary stenosis on fractional flow reserve assessment of intermediate left main

coronary artery disease: human validation. JACC Cardiovasc Interv 2015;8:398–403.

22. Tu S, Westra J, Yang J, et al. Diagnostic Accuracy of Fast Computational Approaches to Derive Fractional Flow Reserve From Diagnostic Coronary Angiography: The International Multicenter FAVOR Pilot Study. JACC Cardiovasc interventions 2016;9: 2024–35.

23. Xu B, Tu S, Qiao S, et al. Diagnostic Accuracy of Angiography-Based Quantitative Flow Ratio Measurements for Online Assessment of Coronary Stenosis. J Am Coll Cardiol 2017;70:3077–87.

24. Biscaglia S, Tebaldi M, Brugaletta S, et al. Prognostic Value of QFR Measured Immediately After Successful Stent Implantation: The International Multicenter Prospective HAWKEYE Study. JACC Cardiovasc interventions 2019;12:2079–88.

25. Tu S, Ding D, Chang Y, et al. Diagnostic accuracy of quantitative flow ratio for assessment of coronary stenosis significance from a single angiographic view: A novel method based on bifurcation fractal law. Catheterization Cardiovasc interventions 2021;1040–7.

26. Hildick-Smith D, de Belder AJ, Cooter N, et al. Randomized trial of simple versus complex drug-eluting stenting for bifurcation lesions: the British Bifurcation Coronary Study: old, new, and evolving strategies. Circulation 2010;121:1235–43.

27. Steigen TK, Maeng M, Wiseth R, et al. Randomized study on simple versus complex stenting of coronary artery bifurcation lesions: the Nordic bifurcation study. Circulation 2006;114:1955–61.

28. Ferenc M, Gick M, Kienzle RP, et al. Randomized trial on routine vs. provisional T-stenting in the treatment of de novo coronary bifurcation lesions. Eur Heart J 2008;29:2859–67.

29. Colombo A, Bramucci E, Sacca S, et al. Randomized study of the crush technique versus provisional side-branch stenting in true coronary bifurcations: the CACTUS (Coronary Bifurcations: Application of the Crushing Technique Using Sirolimus-Eluting Stents) Study. Circulation 2009;119:71–8.

30. Chen SL, Santoso T, Zhang JJ, et al. A randomized clinical study comparing double kissing crush with provisional stenting for treatment of coronary bifurcation lesions: results from the DKCRUSH-II (Double Kissing Crush versus Provisional Stenting Technique for Treatment of Coronary Bifurcation Lesions) trial. J Am Coll Cardiol 2011;57:914–20.

31. Kumsars I, Holm N, Niemelä M, et al. Randomised comparison of provisional side branch stenting versus a two-stent strategy for treatment of true coronary bifurcation lesions involving a large side branch: the Nordic-Baltic Bifurcation Study IV. Open heart 2020;7:e000947.

32. Chen SL, Zhang JJ, Han Y, et al. Double Kissing Crush Versus Provisional Stenting for Left Main Distal Bifurcation Lesions: DKCRUSH-V Randomized Trial. J Am Coll Cardiol 2017;70:2605–17.

33. Hildick-Smith D, Behan M, Lassen J, et al. The EBC TWO Study (European Bifurcation Coronary TWO): A Randomized Comparison of Provisional T-Stenting Versus a Systematic 2 Stent Culotte Strategy in Large Caliber True Bifurcations. Circ Cardiovasc interventions 2016;9.

34. Hildick-Smith D, Egred M, Banning A, et al. The European bifurcation club Left Main Coronary Stent study: a randomized comparison of stepwise provisional vs. systematic dual stenting strategies (EBC MAIN). Eur Heart J 2021;42(37):3829–39.

35. Chen SL, Zhang JJ, Ye F, et al. Study comparing the double kissing (DK) crush with classical crush for the treatment of coronary bifurcation lesions: the DKCRUSH-1 Bifurcation Study with drug-eluting stents. Eur J Clin Invest 2008;38:361–71.

36. Chen SL, Xu B, Han YL, et al. Comparison of double kissing crush versus Culotte stenting for unprotected distal left main bifurcation lesions: results from a multicenter, randomized, prospective DKCRUSH-III study. J Am Coll Cardiol 2013;61: 1482–8.

37. Erglis A, Kumsars I, Niemelä M, et al. Randomized comparison of coronary bifurcation stenting with the crush versus the culotte technique using sirolimus eluting stents: the Nordic stent technique study. Circ Cardiovasc interventions 2009;2:27–34.

38. Ferenc M, Gick M, Comberg T, et al. Culotte stenting vs. TAP stenting for treatment of de-novo coronary bifurcation lesions with the need for side-branch stenting: the Bifurcations Bad Krozingen (BBK) II angiographic trial. Eur Heart J 2016;37: 3399–405.

39. Banning AP, Lassen JF, Burzotta F, et al. Percutaneous coronary intervention for obstructive bifurcation lesions: the 14th consensus document from the European Bifurcation Club. EuroIntervention 2019; 15:90–8.

40. Niemelä M, Kervinen K, Erglis A, et al. Randomized comparison of final kissing balloon dilatation versus no final kissing balloon dilatation in patients with coronary bifurcation lesions treated with main vessel stenting: the Nordic-Baltic Bifurcation Study III. Circulation 2011;123:79–86.

41. Finet G, Derimay F, Motreff P, et al. Comparative Analysis of Sequential Proximal Optimizing Technique Versus Kissing Balloon Inflation Technique in Provisional Bifurcation Stenting: Fractal Coronary Bifurcation Bench Test. JACC Cardiovasc interventions 2015;8:1308–17.

42. Sawaya FJ, Lefèvre T, Chevalier B, et al. Contemporary Approach to Coronary Bifurcation Lesion Treatment. JACC Cardiovasc Interv 2016;9:1861–78.

43. Colombo A, Moses JW, Morice MC, et al. Randomized study to evaluate sirolimus-eluting stents

implanted at coronary bifurcation lesions. Circulation 2004;109:1244–9.

44. Burzotta F, Džavík V, Ferenc M, et al. Technical aspects of the T And small Protrusion (TAP) technique. EuroIntervention 2015;11(Suppl V):V91–5.

45. Chevalier B, Glatt B, Royer T, et al. Placement of coronary stents in bifurcation lesions by the "culotte" technique. Am J Cardiol 1998;82:943–9.

46. Hu F, Tu S, Cai W, et al. Double kissing mini-culotte versus mini-culotte stenting: insights from micro-computed tomographic imaging of bench testing. EuroIntervention 2019;15:465–72.

47. Fan L, Chen L, Luo Y, et al. DK mini-culotte stenting in the treatment of true coronary bifurcation lesions: a propensity score matching comparison with T-provisional stenting. Heart and vessels 2016;31:308–21.

48. Kandzari DE, Gershlick AH, Serruys PW, et al. Outcomes Among Patients Undergoing Distal Left Main Percutaneous Coronary Intervention. Circ Cardiovasc interventions 2018;11:e007007.

49. Chen X, Li X, Zhang JJ, et al. 3-Year Outcomes of the DKCRUSH-V Trial Comparing DK Crush With Provisional Stenting for Left Main Bifurcation Lesions. JACC Cardiovasc Interv 2019;12:1927–37.

50. Chen SL, Xu B, Han YL, et al. Clinical Outcome After DK Crush Versus Culotte Stenting of Distal Left Main Bifurcation Lesions: The 3-Year Follow-Up Results of the DKCRUSH-III Study. JACC Cardiovasc Interv 2015;8:1335–42.

51. Chen SL, Santoso T, Zhang JJ, et al. Clinical Outcome of Double Kissing Crush Versus Provisional Stenting of Coronary Artery Bifurcation Lesions: The 5-Year Follow-Up Results From a Randomized and Multicenter DKCRUSH-II Study (Randomized Study on Double Kissing Crush Technique Versus Provisional Stenting Technique for Coronary Artery Bifurcation Lesions). Circ Cardiovasc interventions 2017;10.

52. Harada Y, Colleran R, Pinieck S, et al. Angiographic and clinical outcomes of patients treated with drug-coated balloon angioplasty for in-stent restenosis after coronary bifurcation stenting with a two-stent technique. EuroIntervention 2017;12:2132–9.

53. Jing Q, Zhao X, Han Y, et al. A drug-eluting Balloon for the trEatment of coronarY bifurcatiON lesions in the side branch: a prospective multicenter ranDomized (BEYOND) clinical trial in China. Chin Med J 2020;133:899–908.

Recent Advances in Antiplatelet Therapy in Complex Percutaneous Coronary Intervention

Alessandro Spirito, MD[1], Peter Cangialosi, MD[1],
Davide Cao, MD, Johny Nicolas, MD,
Roxana Mehran, MD*

KEYWORDS

- Antiplatelet therapy • Complex PCI • Dual antithrombotic therapy • Dual pathway inhibition
- Left main disease

KEY POINTS

- Bleeding risk should be first taken into account when deciding on the antiplatelet strategy in patients undergoing complex PCI.
- Among high bleeding risk patients undergoing complex PCI, DAPT for 1 or 3 months, followed by either aspirin or P2Y12 inhibitor monotherapy should be considered.
- In absence of high bleeding risk, a DAPT duration longer than the period mandated by guidelines seems reasonable in complex PCI patients
- The role of dual pathway inhibition immediately after PCI and DAPT de-escalation needs to be further investigated in the context of patients with complex PCI

INTRODUCTION

Antiplatelet therapy is the cornerstone of secondary cardiovascular prevention after percutaneous coronary intervention (PCI).[1] Improvements in drug-eluting stent (DES) technologies (ie, thinner stent struts, higher polymer biocompatibility, and improved drug release kinetics) and advances in the medical therapy over the last 2 decades have led to changes in current antithrombotic strategies.[1] Current guidelines recommend at least 6 or 12 months of dual antiplatelet therapy (DAPT) after elective PCI or acute coronary syndrome (ACS), respectively. However, DAPT duration should be tailored based on individual ischemic and bleeding risk.[1,2] Over the last several years, novel approaches including DAPT de-escalation, dual pathway inhibition (DPI), and especially a short DAPT duration followed by P2Y12 monotherapy, have been proposed to prevent cardiac ischemic events while minimizing bleeding risk.[3] However, it remains unclear whether specific high-risk patient subsets, such as those undergoing complex PCI, would benefit from such strategies.

Given the growing number of patients undergoing complex PCI,[4,5] it is a priority to define the optimal antiplatelet treatment in this challenging subgroup. Complex PCI intuitively requires a prolonged or more potent antiplatelet therapy, which is, however, associated with a greater risk of bleeding complications. In this review article, we sought to summarize and discuss the current evidence on antiplatelet therapy in patients undergoing complex PCI.

Zena and Michael A. Wiener Cardiovascular Institute Icahn School of Medicine at Mount Sinai, One Gustave L. Levy Place, Box 1030, New York, NY 10029, USA
[1]These authors contributed equally to this work
* Corresponding author. Center for Interventional Cardiovascular Research and Clinical Trials, Icahn School of Medicine at Mount Sinai, One Gustave L. Levy Place, BOX 1030, New York, NY 10029.
E-mail address: Roxana.mehran@mountsinai.org
Twitter: @DrRoxMehran (R.M.)

Intervent Cardiol Clin 11 (2022) 419–428
https://doi.org/10.1016/j.iccl.2022.02.003
2211-7458/22/© 2022 Elsevier Inc. All rights reserved.

DEFINITION OF COMPLEX PERCUTANEOUS CORONARY INTERVENTION

A universal definition of complex PCI is lacking. Complex PCI generally refers to procedures involving complex lesions (eg, long, calcified, and bifurcation lesions, or lesions located in a bypass graft) or requiring advanced techniques (eg, bifurcation stenting, atherectomy), which are associated with an increased risk of major adverse cardiovascular events (MACE).[6–8] Several definitions of complex PCI have been used across different studies, yet the one by Giustino and colleagues[9] remains the most frequently used as a means to distinguish patients at lower or higher risk of ischemic complications.[10] This definition includes bifurcation with 2 stents implanted, ≥ 3 stents implanted, ≥ 3 lesions treated, 3 vessels treated, total stent length greater than 60 mm, or treatment of a chronic total occlusion. Other procedural characteristics, such as the treatment of a lesion located in the left main (LM) artery, in vein grafts, a bifurcation with side branch diameter ≥ 2.5 mm, a lesion length ≥ 30 mm, containing thrombus, or severely calcified lesion requiring coronary atherectomy, have been also used to characterize complex PCI (Fig. 1).[8]

PROLONGED ANTIPLATELET THERAPY

In a patient-level meta-analysis including 9577 patients from 6 randomized controlled trials (RCTs), Giustino and colleagues compared the safety and efficacy of a short- (3 or 6 months) versus long-term (>12 months) DAPT.[9] At a median follow-up of 392 days, among subjects undergoing complex PCI (n = 1680), long-term DAPT was associated with a significant reduction in MACE (a composite of cardiac death, myocardial infarction [MI], definite/probable stent thrombosis [ST]) as compared with short-term DAPT (4.1% vs 6.8%, adjusted hazard ratio [HR]: 0.56; 95% confidence interval [CI]: 0.35–0.89) (Table 1). In contrast, this effect was not observed among those undergoing non-complex PCI (2.9% vs 2.9%, adjusted HR: 1.01, 95% CI: 0.75–1.35). The rates of bleeding events were numerically higher with long-compared with short-term DAPT, although significantly increased only in non-complex PCI (1.9% vs 1.3%; adjusted HR: 1.45, 95% CI: 1.02–2.07) but not in patients with complex PCI (2.6% vs 1.6%, adjusted HR: 1.64, 95% CI: 0.83–3.26). Of note, the benefits of prolonged DAPT seemed to be consistent across the different categories of complex PCI, DES generation, and clinical presentation.

The DAPT randomized trial compared a continuation of DAPT for 18 additional months versus aspirin alone in event-free patients at 1 year after PCI. Among the 3730 patients who underwent complex PCI,[11] based on the study definition (see Table 1), continuation of DAPT was associated with a significant reduction of the composite primary outcome of death, MI, or stroke (4.7% vs 6.3%, HR: 0.72; 95% CI: 0.55–0.96) as well as of MI or ST (2.5% vs 4.5%, HR: 0.55; 95% CI: 0.38–0.79) without a relevant increase in GUSTO moderate/severe

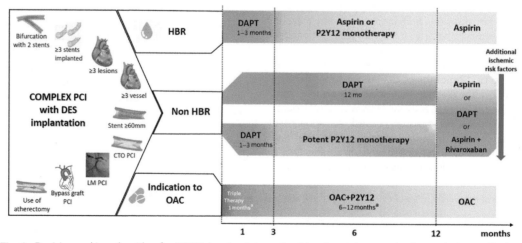

Fig. 1. Decision-making algorithm for DAPT duration integrating bleeding risk, procedural complexity, and indication to oral anticoagulation in patients undergoing complex PCI. PCI, percutaneous coronary intervention; DES, drug-eluting stent; HBR, high bleeding risk; OAC, oral anticoagulation (Vitamin K antagonist or new oral anticoagulant); DAPT, dual antiplatelet therapy; CTO, chronic total occlusion; LM, left main. [a]according to the presence of additional high bleeding risk factors.

Table 1
Key studies assessing the efficacy and safety of antiplatelet therapies in patients undergoing complex PCI without indication to oral anticoagulation

Study Name First Author, Date of publication	Giustino et al., 2016[9]	DAPT Yeh et al., 2017[11]	Costa et al., 2019[12]	GLOBAL LEADERS Serruys et al., 2019[20]	TWILIGHT Dangas et al., 2020[22]	SMART CHOICE Roh et al., 2021[23]	STOPDAPT-2 Yamamoto et al., 2021[21]
Study design	IPD meta-analysis of 6 RCTs	RCT post hoc analysis	IPD meta-analysis of 8 RCTs	RCT post hoc analysis	RCT post hoc analysis	RCT post hoc analysis	RCT post hoc analysis
N° of patients with complex PCI	1680	3730	3118	4570	2342	498	509
Short DAPT duration (months)	3–6	12	1–6	1	3	3	1
Monotherapy following DAPT	Aspirin	Aspirin	Aspirin	Ticagrelor	Ticagrelor	Any oral P2Y12 inhibitor	Clopidogrel or prasugrel
Long DAPT duration (months)	≥12	30	≥12 (followed by aspirin)	12 (followed by aspirin)	15	12	12
P2Y12 inhibitor in DAPT (%)	Clopidogrel (100)	Clopidogrel (68) Prasugrel (32)	Clopidogrel (79.5) Ticagrelor (8.5) Prasugrel (10.0)	Ticagrelor or Clopidogrel (stable CAD)	Ticagrelor (100)	Clopidogrel (77) Ticagrelor (19) Prasugrel (4)	Clopidogrel (60) Prasugrel (40)
ACS (%)	44	42	57	68	65	58	38
2nd gen. DES (%)	87	60	81	68	65	58	38
Complex PCI definition	Giustino criteria[a]	Study specific criteria[b]	Giustino criteria	Giustino criteria	Giustino criteria + additional criteria[c]	Giustino criteria (excluding CTO)	Giustino criteria
Follow-up	392 d	30 mo	24 mo	24 mo	15 mo	12 mo	12 mo
Comparison	Short vs long	Short vs long	Short-long	Short vs long	Short vs long	Short vs long	Short vs long
Ischemic endpoint definition	Cardiac death, MI, definite/probable ST	Death, MI, stroke	MI, definite ST, stroke or TVR	Death or MI	Death, MI or stroke	all-cause death, MI or stroke	CV death, MI, definite ST, stroke

(continued on next page)

Table 1
(continued)

Study Name First Author, Date of publication	Giustino et al., 2016[9]	DAPT Yeh et al., 2017[11]	Costa et al., 2019[12]	GLOBAL LEADERS Serruys et al., 2019[20]	TWILIGHT Dangas et al., 2020[22]	SMART CHOICE Roh et al., 2021[23]	STOPDAPT-2 Yamamoto et al., 2021[21]
Ischemic endpoint: crude rate (%), HR (95% CI)	4.1 vs 6.8 0.56 (0.35–0.89)	4.7 vs 6.3 0.72 (0.55–0.96)	HBR−: −3.86 (−7.71 to +0.06) HBR+: +1.30 (−6.99 to +9.57)	3.51 vs 5.43 0.64 (0.48–0.85)	3.8 vs 4.9 0.77 (0.52–1.15)	3.8 vs 4.2 0.92 (0.38–2.21)	1.7 vs 3.0 0.54 (0.16–1.79)
Bleeding definition	TIMI, BARC or REPLACE	GUSTO Moderate/ severe	TIMI major or minor	BARC 3 or 5	BARC 2, 3 or 5	BARC 2–5	TIMI major or minor
Bleeding: crude rate (%), HR (95% CI)	2.6 vs 1.6 1.64 (0.83–3.26)	2.2 vs 1.6 1.41 (0.87–2.28)	HBR−: +0.28% (−0.46 to +1.26) HBR+: 3.04 (−2.97–8.82)	2.45 vs 2.54 0.97 (0.67–1.40)	4.2 vs 7.7 0.54 (0.38–0.76)	1.9 vs 3.4 0.58 0.19–1.77	0 vs 2.29 -

Abbreviations: IPD, individual patient data; RCT, randomized controlled trial; PCI, percutaneous coronary intervention; DAPT, dual antiplatelet therapy; CAD, coronary artery disease; ACS, acute coronary syndrome; DES, drug-eluting stent; MI, myocardial infarction; ST, stent thrombosis; TVR, target vessel revascularization; CV, cardiovascular; CI, confidence interval; HR, Hazard ratio

[a] Bifurcation with 2 stents implanted, ≥ 3 stents implanted, ≥ 3 lesions treated, 3 vessels treated, total stent length greater than 60 mm or treatment of a chronic total occlusion.
[b] Unprotected left main stented, greater than 2 lesions per vessel, Lesion length greater than 30 mm, Bifurcation lesion with side branch ≥2.5 mm stented, Vein bypass graft stented, Thrombus-containing lesion.
[c] Left main PCI, Vein bypass graft PCI, use of atherectomy device

bleeding (2.2% vs 1.6%, HR: 1.41, 95% CI: 0.87–2.28) (see Table 1). In the non-complex PCI group treated with extended DAPT, ischemic events were lower (death, MI or stroke 4.1% vs 5.5%, HR: 0.74, 95% CI: 0.60–0.91), but bleeding complications significantly higher (2.5% vs 1.4%, HR: 1.78, 95% CI: 1.27–2.50). The authors showed the value of the DAPT score to identify those patients that would benefit the most from an extended treatment duration without incurring bleeding-related harm. The score included procedure-related variables such as the use of a paclitaxel-eluting stent, stent diameter less than 3 mm, and vein graft stent.

In a pooled analysis of 8 RCTs,[12] including 14,963 patients stratified according to PCI complexity and high bleeding risk (HBR) status (defined as PRECISE-DAPT score ≥25), the efficacy and safety of short-term (3 or 6 months) versus long-term (12 or 24 months) DAPT were evaluated. In patients with non-HBR undergoing complex PCI, long-term DAPT reduced ischemic events (a composite of MI, definite ST, stroke or target vessel revascularization [TVR]; absolute risk difference [ARD]: −3.86%; 95% CI: −7.71 to +0.06) without a significant increase in TIMI major or minor bleeding (ARD: +0.28%; 95% CI: −0.46 to +1.26) (see Table 1). Conversely, among patients with HBR, there was no reduction in ischemic complications but rather a higher rate of bleeding events, irrespective of PCI complexity. Of note, although the net clinical benefit of long-term DAPT in patients with non-HBR was numerically higher among those who underwent complex PCI, statistical interaction was only achieved when ACS presentation was included in the definition of complex PCI (P for interaction < 0.001).

These findings suggest that maintaining patients on DAPT for 12 months or longer may be beneficial in the setting of complex PCI, provided that they are not HBR. Moreover, incorporating angiographic with clinical high-risk features seems to allow a better ischemic risk stratification to inform the DAPT regimen (see Fig. 1).

DE-ESCALATION

An unguided or guided DAPT de-escalation may represent an interesting option to prevent effectively ischemic complications in the first weeks after PCI, without increasing long-term bleeding risk. The reduction of net adverse cardiac events (NACE) was consistent across patients with single or multivessel disease or shorter (<40 mm) versus longer (≥40 mm) total stent length in TALOS-AMI[13] and HOST-REDUCE-POLYTECH-ACS.[14] In

another trial assessing a genotype-guided DAPT, NACE were similar between the group of patients undergoing multivessel PCI with genotype-guided and the control arm treated with standard DAPT arm (p for interaction 0.68).[15]

The routine use of such strategies is currently not recommended,[16] and their efficacy and safety on patients undergoing complex PCI remains unknown.

DUAL PATHWAY INHIBITION

In recent years, the concept of DPI, consisting of a synergistical combination of a novel oral anticoagulant (NOAC) with dual or single antiplatelet therapy, has been proposed for post-PCI pharmacologic management.

The APPRAISE study showed that among patients with ACS with high-risk clinical features (44% of those treated with PCI) the addition of apixaban, at a dose of 5 mg twice daily to DAPT increased the number of major bleeding events without a significant reduction in ischemic events as compared with standard DAPT.[17]

The GEMINI-ACS-1 trial[18] examined the effect of rivaroxaban 2.5 mg in association with a P2Y12 inhibitor versus standard DAPT (aspirin plus P2Y12 inhibitor) in 3037 patients with ACS. The experimental group had similar rates of clinically significant bleeding as the traditional aspirin-based DAPT group at 12 months (5% in both). However, the study was underpowered to detect any differences in ischemic events. Additional studies are needed to determine the risk profile of patients with ACS (eg, those undergoing complex PCI) who would benefit the most from low-dose rivaroxaban in addition to P2Y12 inhibition.

The COMPASS trial[19] tested low-dose rivaroxaban 2.5 mg twice-daily plus aspirin 100 mg once-daily (DPI group) versus aspirin 100 mg once-daily alone in patients with established stable cardiovascular disease. In a prespecified subgroup analysis focused on 9862 patients with prior PCI (38% with multivessel PCI), DPI compared with aspirin was associated with a reduction on MACE (4.0% vs 5.5%; HR: 0.74, 95% CI: 0.61–0.88) and mortality (2.5% vs 3.5%; HR: 0.73, 95% CI: 0.58–0.92) at the expense of a higher major bleeding rate (3.3% vs 2.0%; HR: 1.72, 95% CI: 1.34–2.21). No heterogeneity was noted between prior single- and multi-vessel PCI with DPI compared with aspirin alone (P for interaction 0.31). Of note, the addition of a low dose of rivaroxaban on top of aspirin reduced the risk of stroke, a finding that has never been observed in studies assessing the effects of a prolonged DAPT. Nonetheless, there was no statistically significant reduction in MI. Based on these results, a DPI strategy seems reasonable in patients with non-HBR undergoing complex-PCI and well-stabilized CAD (see Fig. 1).

ROLE OF ANTIPLATELET MONOTHERAPY

Several trials have investigated the efficacy and safety of a brief course of DAPT followed by monotherapy with P2Y12 inhibitor as an alternative to standard DAPT.

In a post hoc analysis of the GLOBAL LEADERS trial[20] the experimental regimen of 1 month of DAPT followed by 23 months of ticagrelor monotherapy was compared with 12 months of DAPT followed by 12 months of aspirin monotherapy according to PCI complexity. Among 4570 patients undergoing complex PCI, the experimental compared with the standard regimen significantly reduced the 2-year risk of all-cause death or new Q-wave MI (3.51% vs 5.43%, HR: 0.64; 95% CI: 0.48–0.85) and of a composite of all-cause death, any stroke, any MI, or any revascularization (14.02% vs 17.20%, HR: 0.80; 95% CI: 0.69–0.93), while maintaining a similar risk of BARC type 3 or 5 bleeding (2.45% vs 2.54%, HR: 0.97; 95% CI: 0.67–1.40) (see Table 1). According to the subgroup analysis, this benefit was mainly related to ACS presentation (p for interaction between patients with ACS and stable CAD <0.05).

In a substudy of the STOP-DAPT2 trial,[21] designed to assess the noninferiority of 1 month of DAPT followed by clopidogrel or prasugrel monotherapy versus standard 12-month DAPT, among 509 patients with complex PCI the 12-month risk for the primary composite endpoint (consisting of cardiovascular death, MI, ischemic or hemorrhagic stroke, definite stent thrombosis or major or minor bleeding) was significantly reduced in the monotherapy group as compared with the 12-month DAPT group (1.67% vs 5.32%, adj.HR: 0.30; 95% CI: 0.10–0.92) (see Table 1).

A similar analysis was conducted in the TWILIGHT study,[22] which examined the effects of 3-month DAPT followed by ticagrelor monotherapy for 12 months versus a ticagrelor-based DAPT for 15 months. Among the 2342 patients undergoing complex PCI, ticagrelor monotherapy was associated with significantly lower rates of BARC type 2, 3, or 5 bleeding (4.2% vs 7.7%, ARD: -3.5%, HR: 0.54; 95% CI: 0.38–0.76) without significant differences in the composite ischemic endpoint of death, MI, or stroke (3.8% vs 4.9%, ARD: -1.1%, HR: 0.77; 95% CI: 0.52–

1.15) (see Table 1). Of note, the treatment effects on the ischemic endpoint were consistent between the complex and non-complex patient groups (P for interaction = 0.13).

A post hoc analysis of the SMART-CHOICE trial[23] showed that among 498 patients undergoing complex PCI, P2Y12 inhibitor monotherapy (77% clopidogrel) following 3 months of DAPT was associated with a similar risk of all-cause death, MI, or stroke (3.8% vs 4.2% HR: 0.92, 95% CI: 0.38–2.21) and BARC 2 to 5 (1.9% vs 3.4%, HR: 0.58 95% CI: 0.19–1.77) as compared with standard 12-month DAPT (see Table 1).

In a pooled analysis of STOPDAPT and STOPDAPT-2 ACS trials, there were no differences in the primary outcome of the composite of cardiovascular death, MI, ST, stroke, and TIMI major/minor bleeding between a 1-month DAPT followed by clopidogrel monotherapy versus a 12-month DAPT regimen, and these results seemed to be consistent between patients undergoing a complex (n = 1893) or non-complex PCI (P for interaction = 0.48).[24]

According to these results, monotherapy with a P2Y12 inhibitor, ideally a potent agent, following a short duration of DAPT may represent an optimal treatment even in patients undergoing complex PCI (see Fig. 1).

SPECIFIC COHORTS

The most common definition used for complex PCI[9] does not include the treatment of the LM, a vein bypass graft, or the use of an atherectomy, which are also associated with a higher risk of ischemic complications.[8] LM and vein bypass graft PCI were included in the complex PCI definition of the DAPT trial substudy,[11] but the effects of the antiplatelet regimen for each complex PCI category (eg, PCI involving LM, a vein bypass graft, stent length >40 mm) were not provided. Conversely, in the TWILIGHT complex PCI substudy,[22] the reduction of bleeding without an increase in ischemic complications was consistent across all complex PCI criteria, which included LM, vein bypass graft PCI, and use of an atherectomy device.

In a substudy of the PRODIGY trial,[25] which included 953 patients with LM or proximal left anterior descending artery stenosis, 24- versus 6-month DAPT did not result in a reduction of the composite endpoint of death, MI, or cerebrovascular accident (11.0% vs 11.0%; HR: 0.96; 95% CI: 0.65–1.41, P = .84), but decreased the risk of definite, probable, or possible ST (2.8% vs 5.6%; HR: 0.45; 95% CI: 0.23–0.89, P = .02), regardless of clinical presentation.

However, 24-month DAPT was associated with a higher risk of BARC type 2, 3, or 5 bleeding (8.7% vs 3.5%, HR: 2.51, 95% CI: 1.43–4.42).

In a post hoc analysis of the EXCEL trial,[26] 497 patients with LM PCI and event-free at 1 year received DAPT for 3 additional years, while 136 discontinued DAPT immediately. The long-DAPT compared with the short regimen did not reduce the primary ischemic composite endpoint of death, MI, or stroke (7.9% vs 5.2%, HR: 1.59, 95% CI: 0.69–3.48). There was no difference in the need for blood product transfusion (0.9% vs 1.5%).

Given the limited evidence with antiplatelet strategies for specific categories of complex PCI, it is reasonable to apply the same antiplatelet strategy to these different subsets.

PATIENTS REQUIRING LONG-TERM ANTICOAGULATION

Antiplatelet therapy for patients requiring long-term anticoagulation undergoing complex PCI is challenging. Oral anticoagulation significantly increases the bleeding risk and, accordingly, was included as a major HBR criterion by the ARC consensus.[27] Subgroup analyses of 2 large randomized trials provided relevant insights about the optimal treatment in this subgroup of patients.

In a substudy of the PIONEER AF-PCI,[28] patients with atrial fibrillation (AF) undergoing PCI were randomized to rivaroxaban 15 mg once daily plus a P2Y12 inhibitor (93% clopidogrel) for 12 months or to standard therapy with a dose-adjusted vitamin K antagonist plus DAPT (96% aspirin plus clopidogrel) for 1, 6, or 12 months (16%, 35%, and 49%, respectively). Sixty-six percent of subjects received a DES, and 52% presented with ACS. Compared with warfarin, the rivaroxaban regimen reduced TIMI major or minor bleeding or bleeding requiring medical attention without increasing ischemic complications (a composite of death from cardiovascular causes, MI or stroke) consistently after stratification according to the presence of multivessel disease, bifurcation lesion, thrombus, stent length or number of stents implanted. Of note, the study was underpowered for ischemic outcomes, which limits the ability to draw any definitive conclusion regarding its safety.

RE-DUAL PCI randomly assigned patients with AF undergoing PCI to dual antithrombotic therapy (DAT) with a P2Y12 inhibitor (87% clopidogrel) and dabigatran 110 or 150 mg for 12 months or to triple therapy, consisting of warfarin, aspirin, and a P2Y12 inhibitor (90%

clopidogrel) for at least 1 month in patients treated with bare metal stent and 3 months in those receiving a DES (82%). Half of the included patients had an ACS. Among the 270 patients with at least one criterion of procedural complexity (defined as in the DAPT trial[11]) there was a trend toward a reduction of major or clinically relevant non-major bleeding events according to the ISTH classification with dabigatran 110 or 150 mg dual therapy as compared with warfarin triple therapy (Dabigatran 110 mg vs Warfarin: 15.1% vs 27.8%, HR: 0.48, 95% CI: 0.35–0.65; Dabigatran 150 mg vs Warfarin: 13.8% vs 25.8%, HR: 0.48, 95% CI: 0.22–1.02) without an increase of the composite ischemic outcome of death, MI, stroke, systemic embolism, or unplanned PCI or coronary artery bypass graft surgery (Dabigatran 110 mg vs Warfarin: 15.1% vs 14.4%, HR: 1.01, 95% CI: 0.48–2.14; Dabigatran 150 mg vs Warfarin: 10% vs 13.6% HR: 0.74, 95% CI: 0.29–1.93).[29]

Overall, these results support the use of NOAC plus P2Y12 monotherapy to manage patients with a history of AF undergoing complex PCI, but in the context of the relatively small sample analyzed, additional studies are needed to confirm these results. Moreover, given the modest and not statistically significant increase of stent thrombosis in the aspirin-free arm,[30,31] caution is needed for very early DAT in this subgroup of patients (see Fig. 1).

FUTURE PERSPECTIVES

Several randomized controlled trials on antithrombotic therapies after PCI are ongoing.[32] Among them, SMART ATTEMPT (NCT04014803) is examining the effect on MACE of a 12-month DAPT with prasugrel versus 12-month DAPT with clopidogrel in patients undergoing elective complex PCI with DES. The TAILORED-CHIP (NCT03465644) is evaluating the impact on NACE of a 6-month DAPT with low-dose ticagrelor followed by 6-month clopidogrel monotherapy versus 12-month DAPT with clopidogrel in high-risk patients undergoing complex PCI.

SUMMARY

Complex PCI increases the risk of ischemic complications proportionally to the number of angiographic high-risk features. In patients undergoing complex PCI, bleeding risk should be first considered when deciding the antiplatelet strategy. Among patients with HBR undergoing complex PCI, DAPT for 1 or 3 months, followed by either aspirin or P2Y12 inhibitor monotherapy should be considered. In non-HBR individuals, a DAPT duration longer than the period mandated by guidelines or 1 to 3-month DAPT followed by monotherapy with P2Y12 inhibitor, ideally one that is potent, seems reasonable after complex PCI regardless of the clinical presentation (ACS or stable ischemic heart disease). Extension of DAPT beyond 12 months can be considered if the treatment was well tolerated and correction in presence of additional clinical risk factors for ischemic complications. Alternatively, secondary prevention can be achieved with aspirin and low-dose rivaroxaban. The role of DPI immediately after PCI and DAPT de-escalation needs to be further investigated in the context of patients with complex PCI.

In patients with chronic indication to oral anticoagulation undergoing complex PCI, dual therapy which includes a P2Y12 inhibitor, seems to be the best option to reduce bleeding events without increasing ischemic complications and aspirin should be discontinued no later than 1-month post-PCI.

CLINICS CARE POINTS

- Bleeding risk should be first taken into account when deciding on the antiplatelet strategy in patients undergoing complex PCI.

- Among high bleeding risk patients undergoing complex PCI, DAPT for 1 or 3 months, followed by either aspirin or P2Y12 inhibitor monotherapy should be considered.

- In absence of high bleeding risk, a DAPT duration longer than the period mandated by guidelines or 1 to 3-month DAPT followed by a P2Y12 inhibitor monotherapy, ideally a potent agent, seems reasonable in patients with complex PCI with acute or chronic coronary syndrome.

- Extending DAPT beyond 12 months or a regimen with aspirin and a low dose of rivaroxaban, may be considered if the antiplatelet therapy was well tolerated and in the presence of additional high-ischemic risk features.

- The role of dual pathway inhibition immediately after PCI and DAPT de-escalation needs to be further investigated in the context of patients with complex PCI

- In patients on chronic oral anticoagulation undergoing complex PCI, aspirin should be discontinued no later than 1-month post-PCI and dual therapy with a P2Y12 inhibitor continued for at least 6 months.

DISCLOSURE

Dr. R. Mehran reports institutional research grants from Abbott, Abiomed, Applied Therapeutics, ARENA, AstraZeneca, Bayer, Biosensors, Singapore, Boston Scientific, Bristol-Myers Squibb, CardiaWave, CellAegis, CERC, France, Chiesi, Concept Medical, CSL Behring, DSI, Insel Gruppe AG, Medtronic, Novartis Pharmaceuticals, OrbusNeich, Philips, Transverse Medical, Zoll; personal fees from ACC, Boston Scientific, California Institute for Regenerative Medicine (CIRM), Cine-Med Research, Janssen, WebMD, SCAI; consulting fees paid to the institution from Abbott, Abiomed, AM-Pharma, Alleviant Medical, Bayer, Beth Israel Deaconess, CardiaWave, CeloNova, Chiesi, Concept Medical, DSI, Duke University, Idorsia Pharmaceuticals, Medtronic, Novartis, Philips; Equity less than 1% in Applied Therapeutics, Elixir Medical, STEL, CONTROLRAD (spouse); Scientific Advisory Board for AMA, Biosensors (spouse). Dr A. Spirito received a research grant from the Swiss National Science Foundation (SNSF), Switzerland. The other authors have nothing to disclose.

REFERENCES

1. Valgimigli M, Bueno H, Byrne RA, et al. 2017 ESC focused update on dual antiplatelet therapy in coronary artery disease developed in collaboration with EACTS: The Task Force for dual antiplatelet therapy in coronary artery disease of the European Society of Cardiology (ESC) and of the European Association for Cardio-Thoracic Surgery (EACTS). Eur Heart J 2018;39(3):213–60.

2. Levine GN, Bates ER, Bittl JA, et al. ACC/AHA Guideline Focused Update on Duration of Dual Antiplatelet Therapy in Patients With Coronary Artery Disease: A Report of the American College of Cardiology/American Heart Association Task Force on Clinical Practice Guidelines: An Update of the 2011 ACCF/AHA/SCAI Guideline for Percutaneous Coronary Intervention, 2011 ACCF/AHA Guideline for Coronary Artery Bypass Graft Surgery, 2012 ACC/AHA/ACP/AATS/PCNA/SCAI/STS Guideline for the Diagnosis and Management of Patients With Stable Ischemic Heart Disease, 2013 ACCF/AHA Guideline for the Management of ST-Elevation Myocardial Infarction, 2014 AHA/ACC Guideline for the Management of Patients With Non-ST-Elevation Acute Coronary Syndromes, and 2014 ACC/AHA Guideline on Perioperative Cardiovascular Evaluation and Management of Patients Undergoing Noncardiac Surgery. Circulation 2016;134(10):e123–55.

3. Giacoppo D, Matsuda Y, Fovino LN, et al. Short dual antiplatelet therapy followed by P2Y12 inhibitor monotherapy vs. prolonged dual antiplatelet therapy after percutaneous coronary intervention with second-generation drug-eluting stents: a systematic review and meta-analysis of randomized clinical trials. Eur Heart J 2021;42(4):308–19.

4. Bortnick AE, Epps KC, Selzer F, et al. Five-year follow-up of patients treated for coronary artery disease in the face of an increasing burden of co-morbidity and disease complexity (from the NHLBI Dynamic Registry). Am J Cardiol 2014; 113(4):573–9.

5. Werner N, Nickenig G, Sinning JM. Complex PCI procedures: challenges for the interventional cardiologist. Clin Res Cardiol 2018;107(Suppl 2):64–73.

6. Stefanini GG, Serruys PW, Silber S, et al. The impact of patient and lesion complexity on clinical and angiographic outcomes after revascularization with zotarolimus- and everolimus-eluting stents: a substudy of the RESOLUTE All Comers Trial (a randomized comparison of a zotarolimus-eluting stent with an everolimus-eluting stent for percutaneous coronary intervention). J Am Coll Cardiol 2011; 57(22):2221–32.

7. Wilensky RL, Selzer F, Johnston J, et al. Relation of percutaneous coronary intervention of complex lesions to clinical outcomes (from the NHLBI Dynamic Registry). Am J Cardiol 2002;90(3):216–21.

8. Genereux P, Giustino G, Redfors B, et al. Impact of percutaneous coronary intervention extent, complexity and platelet reactivity on outcomes after drug-eluting stent implantation. Int J Cardiol 2018;268:61–7.

9. Giustino G, Chieffo A, Palmerini T, et al. Efficacy and Safety of Dual Antiplatelet Therapy After Complex PCI. J Am Coll Cardiol 2016;68(17):1851–64.

10. Capodanno D. Antiplatelet strategies for complex PCI. EuroIntervention 2019;15(11):e939–42.

11. Yeh RW, Kereiakes DJ, Steg PG, et al. Lesion Complexity and Outcomes of Extended Dual Antiplatelet Therapy After Percutaneous Coronary Intervention. J Am Coll Cardiol 2017;70(18): 2213–23.

12. Costa F, Van Klaveren D, Feres F, et al. Dual Antiplatelet Therapy Duration Based on Ischemic and Bleeding Risks After Coronary Stenting. J Am Coll Cardiol 2019;73(7):741–54.

13. Kim CJ, Park MW, Kim MC, et al. Unguided de-escalation from ticagrelor to clopidogrel in stabilised patients with acute myocardial infarction undergoing percutaneous coronary intervention (TALOS-AMI): an investigator-initiated, open-label, multicentre, non-inferiority, randomised trial. Lancet 2021;398(10308):1305–16.

14. Kim HS, Kang J, Hwang D, et al. Prasugrel-based de-escalation of dual antiplatelet therapy after percutaneous coronary intervention in patients with acute coronary syndrome (HOST-REDUCE-POLYTECH-ACS): an open-label, multicentre, non-inferiority randomised trial. Lancet 2020; 396(10257):1079–89.

15. Claassens DMF, Vos GJA, Bergmeijer TO, et al. A Genotype-Guided Strategy for Oral P2Y12 Inhibitors in Primary PCI. N Engl J Med 2019;381(17): 1621–31.

16. Sibbing D, Aradi D, Alexopoulos D, et al. Updated Expert Consensus Statement on Platelet Function and Genetic Testing for Guiding P2Y12 Receptor Inhibitor Treatment in Percutaneous Coronary Intervention. JACC Cardiovasc Interv 2019;12(16): 1521–37.

17. Alexander JH, Lopes RD, James S, et al. Apixaban with antiplatelet therapy after acute coronary syndrome. N Engl J Med 2011;365(8):699–708.

18. Ohman EM, Roe MT, Steg PG, et al. Clinically significant bleeding with low-dose rivaroxaban versus aspirin, in addition to P2Y12 inhibition, in acute coronary syndromes (GEMINI-ACS-1): a double-blind, multicentre, randomised trial. Lancet 2017; 389(10081):1799–808.

19. Bainey KR, Welsh RC, Connolly SJ, et al. Rivaroxaban Plus Aspirin Versus Aspirin Alone in Patients With Prior Percutaneous Coronary Intervention (COMPASS-PCI). Circulation 2020;141(14):1141–51.

20. Serruys PW, Takahashi K, Chicharoen P, et al. Impact of long-term ticagrelor monotherapy following 1-month dual antiplatelet therapy in patients who underwent complex percutaneous coronary intervention: insights from the Global Leaders trial. Eur Heart J 2019;40(31):2595–604.

21. Yamamoto K, Watanabe H, Morimoto T, et al. Very Short Dual Antiplatelet Therapy After Drug-Eluting Stent Implantation in Patients Who Underwent Complex Percutaneous Coronary Intervention: Insight From the STOPDAPT-2 Trial. Circ Cardiovasc Interv 2021;14(5):e010384.

22. Dangas G, Baber U, Sharma S, et al. Ticagrelor With or Without Aspirin After Complex PCI. J Am Coll Cardiol 2020;75(19):2414–24.

23. Roh JW, Hahn JY, Oh JH, et al. P2Y12 inhibitor monotherapy in complex percutaneous coronary intervention: A post-hoc analysis of SMART-CHOICE randomized clinical trial. Cardiol J 2021. https://doi.org/10.5603/CJ.a2021.0101.

24. Obayashi Y YK. STOPDAPT-2 total cohort: pooled results from two randomized controlled trials of clopidogrel monotherapy after 1-month DAPT following PCI, and subgroup analyses by ACS presentation, HBR, and complex PCI. Presented at: TCT 2021. Orlando, FL. November 5, 2021.

25. Costa F, Adamo M, Ariotti S, et al. Left main or proximal left anterior descending coronary artery disease location identifies high-risk patients

deriving potentially greater benefit from prolonged dual antiplatelet therapy duration. EuroIntervention 2016;11(11):e1222–30.

26. Brener SJ, Serruys PW, Morice MC, et al. Optimal Duration of Dual Antiplatelet Therapy After Left Main Coronary Stenting. J Am Coll Cardiol 2018; 72(17):2086–7.

27. Urban P, Mehran R, Colleran R, et al. Defining High Bleeding Risk in Patients Undergoing Percutaneous Coronary Intervention. Circulation 2019;140(3): 240–61.

28. Kerneis M, Gibson CM, Chi G, et al. Effect of Procedure and Coronary Lesion Characteristics on Clinical Outcomes Among Atrial Fibrillation Patients Undergoing Percutaneous Coronary Intervention: Insights From the PIONEER AF-PCI Trial. JACC Cardiovasc Interv 2018;11(7):626–34.

29. Berry NC, Mauri L, Steg PG, et al. Effect of Lesion Complexity and Clinical Risk Factors on the Efficacy and Safety of Dabigatran Dual Therapy Versus Warfarin Triple Therapy in Atrial Fibrillation After Percutaneous Coronary Intervention: A Subgroup Analysis From the REDUAL PCI Trial. Circ Cardiovasc Interv 2020;13(4):e008349.

30. Lopes RD, Hong H, Harskamp RE, et al. Optimal Antithrombotic Regimens for Patients With Atrial Fibrillation Undergoing Percutaneous Coronary Intervention: An Updated Network Meta-analysis. JAMA Cardiol 2020;5(5):582–9.

31. Capodanno D, Di Maio M, Greco A, et al. Safety and Efficacy of Double Antithrombotic Therapy With Non-Vitamin K Antagonist Oral Anticoagulants in Patients With Atrial Fibrillation Undergoing Percutaneous Coronary Intervention: A Systematic Review and Meta-Analysis. J Am Heart Assoc 2020;9(16):e017212.

32. Cao D, Chandiramani R, Chiarito M, et al. Evolution of antithrombotic therapy in patients undergoing percutaneous coronary intervention: a 40-year journey. Eur Heart J 2021;42(4):339–51.

In-Stent Restenosis

Kenji Kawai, MD[a], Renu Virmani, MD[a], Aloke V. Finn, MD[a,b],*

KEYWORDS

- Bare-metal stent • Drug-eluting stent • Neoatherosclerosis • Intravascular imaging
- Drug-coated balloon

KEY POINTS

- The 2 main biological mechanisms of ISR are neointimal hyperplasia and neoatherosclerosis.
- Impaired endothelial function is important in the pathogenesis of neoatherosclerosis, which develops more slowly with drug-eluting stents compared with bare-metal stents and can lead to acute coronary syndromes.
- Coronary angiography and computed tomography angiography are modalities that allow for morphologic evaluation of ISR, whereas intravascular imaging such as intravascular ultrasound and optical coherence tomography are modalities that can be used to evaluate the nature and potential causes of the ISR lesion.
- Drug-coated balloons are a treatment for ISR that avoids stenting, but evidence for their use compared to stent reimplantation is still controversial, and the choice should be based on patient background and lesion morphology.

INTRODUCTION

Thirty years have already passed since stents were first introduced as a therapeutic device for coronary artery disease. In comparison to bare-metal stents (BMSs), drug-eluting stents (DESs) significantly reduced the risk of in-stent restenosis (ISR) and the need for target lesion revascularization (TLR) by suppressing neointimal proliferation after the stent implantation. However, significant drawbacks of metallic stents remain, including the biocompatibility standpoint of metallic stents. Moreover, and perhaps related, there remains a long-term risk of ISR, even with the newest devices available today. According to the National Cardiovascular Data Registry (NCDR), the number of percutaneous coronary intervention (PCI) for ISR appears to be increasing every year, with approximately 10% of PCI performed in the United States being for this indication.[1–3] As the pathology of stent-specific tissue responses has been increasingly understood, treatment strategies for ISR have also improved. Although newer developments, such as the introduction of drug-coated balloons (DCBs), have offered new treatment options for ISR, the issues surrounding ISR and its treatment have not been completely overcome. This article reviews the pathophysiology as well as pathologic and clinical data regarding ISR and its treatment.

DEFINITION OF IN-STENT RESTENOSIS

Angiographic In-Stent Restenosis

ISR is defined as an angiographic diameter stenosis of 50% or more in a segment of the stent or a 5 mm segment adjacent to the stent.[4,5] Mehran and colleagues classified angiographic ISR into 4 morphologic patterns, based on lesion length, lesion location, and thrombosis in myocardial infarction (TIMI) flow. This classification predicts the risk of revascularization after the stent implantation, with higher grades indicating an increased risk of recurrent ISR and TLR[4] (Box 1). This classification was generated with respect to BMS-ISR primarily, but this risk prediction is adaptive for DES-ISR as well.[5] When the American College of Cardiology/American Heart Association (AHA) lesion

---

[a] CVPath Institute, 19 Firstfield Road, Gaithersburg, MD 20878, USA; [b] University of Maryland, School of Medicine, 22 South Greene Street, Baltimore, MD 21201, USA
* Corresponding author. 19 Firstfield Road, MD, 20878.
E-mail address: afinn@cvpath.org

Intervent Cardiol Clin 11 (2022) 429–443
https://doi.org/10.1016/j.iccl.2022.02.005

Box 1
Definitions and classification of restenosis

- Angiographic Restenosis and Classification
  - Diameter stenosis ≥50%
  - Type 1
    - Focal: ≤10 mm in length
    - 1A: Articulation or gap
    - 1B: Margin
    - 1C: Focal body
    - 1D: Multifocal
  - Type 2
    - Diffuse: greater than 10 mm intrastent
  - Type 3
    - Proliferative: greater than 10 mm extending beyond the stent margins
  - Type 4
    - Total occlusion: restenotic lesions with TIMI flow grade of 0
- Clinical Restenosis: Assessed Objectively as Requirement for Ischemia-Driven Repeat Revascularization
  - Diameter stenosis ≥50% and one of the following:
    - Positive history of recurrent angina pectoris, presumably related to target vessel
    - Objective signs of ischemia at rest (ECG changes) or during exercise test (or equivalent), presumably related to target vessel
    - Abnormal results of any invasive functional diagnostic test (eg, coronary flow velocity reserve, FFR <0.80); IVUS minimum cross-sectional area less than 4 mm^2 (and <6.0 mm^2 for left main stem) has been found to correlate with abnormal FFR and need for subsequent TLR.[9–11]
    - TLR with diameter stenosis ≥70% even in absence of the aforementioned ischemic signs or symptoms

Abbreviations: ECG, electrocardiography; FFR, fractional flow reserve; IVUS, intravascular ultrasound; MI, myocardial infarction; TIMI, thrombolysis in myocardial infarction; TLR, target lesion revascularization.
Permission from Ref.[8]

classification, the most widely used angiographic lesion morphology classification for de-novo lesions, is applied to DES-ISR, higher grade (B2-C) lesions are not only associated with suboptimal results in the acute treatment phase but also with higher rates of restenosis and adverse long-term clinical outcomes.[6]

Clinical In-Stent Restenosis

The definition of clinical restenosis was proposed by the Academic Research Consortium and is defined as the necessity for revascularization based on evidence of ischemia. This definition involves both an assessment of luminal stenosis and the clinical background of the patient (see Box 1).[7] The clinical definition of ISR includes a diameter stenosis of more than 50% with recurrent symptoms or ischemia, or a lumen diameter stenosis of more than 70% without clinical symptoms.[8] The most common clinical evidence of angina includes electrocardiography (ECG) changes indicating ischemia. For intermediate lesions on angiography, fractional flow reserve (FFR) reflecting coronary hemodynamics or intravascular imaging assessing the morphology can provide a diagnosis of myocardial ischemia. Clinical criteria include an FFR of less than 0.80 and a minimal intravascular ultrasound (IVUS) cross-sectional area of less than 4 mm^2 (6 mm^2 for the left main coronary artery).[9–11]

As for other types of ISR, recurrent ISR is defined as the failure of a stented segment with at least 2 prior revascularization procedures.[12] Resistant ISR is defined as recurrent ISR despite conventional multidisciplinary therapy and recurrent within 3-12 months of the last treatment, despite conventional multidisciplinary treatment strategies.[13]

ETIOLOGY

ISR mostly occurs between 3 and 20 months after stenting.[8,14] The reported incidence of ISR varies depending on the stent type. For BMS, it ranges from 16% to 44%, but with the introduction of DES, the frequency of ISR has decreased to 3% to 20%.[15,16] Second-generation stents, because of their improved device designs, have a lower incidence of death and myocardial infarction compared with first-generation DES. Newer generation DES, with improved stent designs, have reduced the incidence of ISR to 5% to 10%.[17–20] However, delayed healing, chronic inflammation, and development of neoatherosclerosis are more common after the DES implantation, and ISR specifically caused by these factors is more common in first- and second-generation DES than in BMS.[1] In addition, approximately 50% of ISR patients have acute coronary syndromes, of which non-ST segment elevation myocardial infarction occurs in 18.7% and ST-segment elevation myocardial infarction in 8.5%.[1,3,21]

The incidence and prevalence of resistant ISR (R-ISR) are unclear. In one large retrospective study, the incidence of R-ISR 10 months after the most recent revascularization procedure was 1.4%.[22] In addition, the onset of R-ISR presented later in the first-generation DES than in the second-generation DES, and the morphologic features on angiography showed that the majority of R-ISR lesions had a focal pattern.[22]

RISK FACTORS

Predictors of ISR include diabetes mellitus, complex lesions (B2/C), small vessels, long stents, and stent underexpansion, and these factors are similar for postimplantation of DES and BMS.[8,23–25] The predictors of ISR are classified into 3 categories, patient-related, lesion-related, and procedural device-related factors (Table 1).[26] As minimal vessel diameter after implantation is an important factor contributing to restenosis, it is important to obtain optimal angiographic results in the acute phase after DES implantation. An intravascular imaging study reported the optimal minimum stent area (MSA) to prevent the occurrence of ISR after stent implantation. The cut-off value of MSA to prevent ISR was 6.4-6.5 mm^2 for BMS, whereas 5.0-5.7 mm^2 for DES.[27–30] Although DES has a smaller MSA cutoff compared with BMS, a smaller stent area can be a risk factor for ISR for both types of stents. In addition, a recent report suggests that autoimmune diseases, insulin-dependent diabetes mellitus, rheumatoid arthritis, systemic lupus erythematosus, antiphospholipid-antibodies syndrome, inflammatory bowel diseases, and Hashimoto's thyroiditis are all risk factors for ISR.[31]

MECHANISM AND CHARACTERISTICS OF IN-STENT RESTENOSIS

The procedure of stent placement into a stenotic lesion involves balloon dilatation to place the stent in close apposition to the arterial wall. As a result, the vessel wall layer containing the plaque is stretched.[32,33] The trigger for ISR is a mechanical vascular injury caused by the balloon-expanded stent itself. Because arterial vessels contain an abundance of elastic fibers, they contribute recoil properties after balloon dilatation.[34] Recoil occurs seconds to minutes after balloon dilatation. Mechanical stretching, endothelial injury, subintimal hemorrhage, and inflammatory responses play an important role, triggering a cascade of several proliferative processes. The complex process of inflammation and repair may continue for weeks, months, or even years in the case of DES-ISR. The major mechanisms of ISR are neointimal hyperplasia and neoatherosclerosis.[35] Calcified nodules have been also reported as an important cause of recurrent ISR.[36–38]

General Mechanism
Intimal and medial injury cause complex inflammatory responses, leading to significant neointimal proliferation via multiple mechanisms.[33] Pathology studies have shown a positive correlation between medial disruption caused by stenting and the degree of neointimal proliferation.[39]

First, vessel wall injury from the delivered stent attracts inflammatory cells (neutrophils and monocytes). Then, adhesion molecules such as intercellular adhesion molecule-1, vascular cell adhesion molecule-1, and MHC class II are activated, exacerbating the accumulation of inflammatory cells. Inflammatory mediators and growth factors derived from activated inflammatory cells (interleukins,

Table 1 Risk factors of in-stent restenosis		
Patient-Related Factors	**Lesion-Related Factors**	**Procedural and Device-Related Factors**
• Diabetes mellitus • Chronic renal insufficiency • Age • Gender • Hypertension • Genetic variant • Drug resistance • Hypersensitivity reaction	• Severe calcification • Bifurcation • Diffuse long lesion • Small vessel • Ostial lesion	• Underexpansion • Stent fracture • Overlapping • Geographic miss • Stent gap • Nonuniform drug elution/deposition • Polymer peering • Residual uncovered atherosclerotic plaques

[1]Reproduced with permission from Ref.[26]

tumor necrosis factor, monocyte chemotactic protein-1, platelet-derived growth factor, basic fibroblast growth factor, heparin-binding epidermal growth factor, etc) promote the production of extracellular matrix (ECM). These also promote migration and proliferation of smooth muscle cells (SMCs) from the media, which eventually leads to neointimal hyperplasia.[26,40–42] Thus, the process of neointimal proliferation is a vascular healing process, in which a variety of coagulation and inflammatory factors and cells stimulate vascular smooth muscle cell (VSMC) proliferation and ECM formation in the injured area.[32]

Redistribution and hyperplasia of SMCs lead to lumen loss. Early ISR lesions are histologically composed of mostly proliferative-rich SMCs and a proteoglycan-rich ECM. Over time, the ECM is replaced with type III and type I collagen.[43] This cellular shift leads to a reduction in the morphology of the lesion, resulting in a relative decrease in late lumen loss. This process occurs over a period of 6 months to 3 years.

Different Characteristics of In-Stent Restenosis Between Bare-Metal Stents and Drug-Eluting Stents

The histology of the neointima in BMS-ISR is characterized as a diffuse pattern with a predominance of VSMC and less ECM. The incidence of BMS-ISR reaches a peak at 3 to 6 months after stent implantation and continues to be relatively stable at 1 year.[35] The neointima of BMS-ISR is hypercellular and enriched in type III collagen and proteoglycans (such as versican and hyaluronic acid) for up to 18 months, after which cellularity and ECM decrease and are replaced by type I collagen (Table 2).

Implanted DESs release localized antiproliferative agents, resulting in delayed vessel wall healing with chronic fibrin deposition, incomplete neointimal formation, and chronic inflammation. This process prevents excessive neointimal hyperplasia after DES implantation and can minimize the incidence of ISR compared with BMS.[44,45] On the other hand, in DES-ISR, hypersensitivity to polymers and drugs, local inflammation, and delayed healing are the main factors in neointimal formation.[46] There are significant differences between BMS-ISR and DES-ISR with regard to the onset period, morphologic features, the underlying matrix, and the reaction to intervention.[5] The morphology of DES-ISR commonly manifests on angiography as a focal pattern (pattern I), which usually includes a stent edge.[47] The histologic features of DES-ISR are mainly composed of ECM deposition and less cellularity.[48] Previous studies have indicated an association between matrix metalloproteinases and the occurrence of DES-ISR.[49,50]

The temporal patterns of BMS-neointimal formation show late neointimal regression with enlarged lumen, whereas DES-neointimal formation shows no significant morphologic

Table 2 Comparison of principal features of restenotic tissue after bare-metal and drug-eluting stent implantation		
	Bare-Metal Stent Restenosis	**Drug-Eluting Stent Restenosis**
Imaging features		
Angiographic morphology	Diffuse pattern more common	Focal pattern more common
Optical coherence tomography tissue properties	Homogeneous, high-signal band most common	Layered structure or heterogeneous most common
Time course of late luminal loss	Late loss maximal by 6–8 mo	Ongoing late loss out to 5 y
Histopathological features		
Smooth muscle cellularity	Rich	Hypocellular
Proteoglycan content	Moderate	High
Peristrut fibrin and inflammation	Occasional	Frequent
Complete endothelialization	3–6 mo	Up to 48 mo
Thrombus present	Occasional	Occasional
Neoatherosclerosis	Relatively infrequent, late	Relatively frequent, accelerated course

Permission from Ref.[5]

regression of the neointima in the chronic phase.[51,52] Neointimal properties of DES-ISR are characterized by the earlier and more frequent occurrence of neoatherosclerosis than in BMS-ISR patients.[5] As a reflection of this characteristic, in BMS-ISR, IVUS is mainly presented with homogeneous, high-signal tissue echoes, whereas DES-ISR commonly shows a layered pattern with a heterogeneous tissue composition[53] (Fig. 1). However, there is still

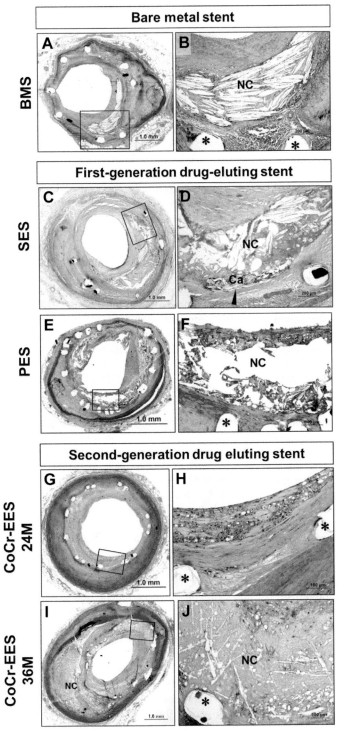

Fig. 1. (*A*, *B*) Low- and high-power images of fibroatheroma within a BMS. (*C*, *D*) Low- and high-power images of fibroatheroma with intraplaque hemorrhage and fragmented calcification (Ca, *arrowheads*) within an SES. (*E*, *F*) Low- and high-power images of thin-cap fibroatheroma within a paclitaxel-eluting stent (PES). (*G*, *H*) Low- and high-power images of fibroatheroma within a cobalt-chromium everolimus-eluting stent (CoCr-EES), which show foamy macrophage accumulation within the neointima 24 months after the implantation. (*I*, *J*) Low- and high-power images of fibroatheroma within a CoCr-EES 36 months after the implantation. *Stent strut. NC, necrotic core. (*A–F*) *Reproduced with permission from Otsuka and colleagues.*[57] (*G–J*) *Reproduced with permission from Otsuka and colleagues.*[108]

controversy regarding the precise mechanisms of DES-ISR, which are not fully understood. It is possible that multiple biological, genetic, mechanical, and technical factors may contribute to DES-ISR.

NEOATHEROSCLEROSIS
General Characteristics of Neoatherosclerosis

After BMS or DES implantation, the development of new atherosclerosis within the neointima of the stented segment is called neoatherosclerosis, which is not only another important mechanism of late stent failure such as late ISR but is also associated with late stent thrombosis.[54] Although neointimal hyperplasia is mainly composed of proteoglycan matrix, SMCs, and interstitial collagen,[55] neoatherosclerosis is characterized by the accumulation of lipid-laden foamy macrophages, necrotic core formation, thin cap fibroatheroma, in-stent plaque rupture, and calcified nodules within the stent, with a variety of these phenotypes seen within the neointima.[36,56,57] In general, the definition of neoatherosclerosis is not dependent on the presence or absence of a necrotic core.[54,57]

Although neoatherosclerotic changes are seen in both BMS and DES, the overall incidence and onset of neoatherosclerosis differ between BMS and DES. In BMS, restenosis with neoatherosclerosis is mainly observed after more than 3 years, with a rate of 38%. In DES, neoatherosclerosis is observed much earlier. In a pathologic analysis of stents with a duration of implant greater than 1 and ≤3 years we conducted, the prevalence of neoatherosclerosis was 48% in second-generation DES versus 6% in BMS.[57] The occurrence of neoatherosclerosis is thought to be related to the presence of antiproliferative agents.[54,58-61] In native coronary arteries without stenting, the progression of atherosclerosis takes decades for the initial lesion to form. This is initiated by the infiltration of macrophage foam cells in the plaque, causing it to develop into vulnerable plaque, such as thin cap fibroatheroma or plaque rupture. However, the course of neoatherosclerosis is characterized by rapid progression after both BMS and DES implantation.

Mechanisms of Neoatherosclerosis

Traditional mTOR inhibitors such as sirolimus or its analogs released from DES increase intracellular calcium levels through the pharmacologic displacement of FKBP12, a ubiquitous, cytosolic 12-KD FK506-binding protein and key stabilizing component of ryanodine (RyR2) intracellular calcium release channels. Increased intracellular calcium activates protein kinase C-alpha, which leads to dissociation of p120-catenin (p120) from VE-cadherin, an important adherens junctional protein responsible for endothelial barrier function.[26,62]

Essentially, a healthy vascular endothelium has the role of preventing the infiltration of leukocytes and platelet aggregation. After stent implantation, immature endothelium in the stented segment has impaired intercellular junctions, leading to further development of atherosclerosis due to the invasion of lipoproteins and monocytes into the subendothelium with decreased expression of antithrombotic agents, decreased nitric oxide production, and impaired barrier function. Endothelial dysfunction covering the stent segment is one factor that contributes to more accelerated neoatherosclerosis, especially in DES as compared with BMS. The accumulation of lipids and foamy macrophages has been associated with the development of DES-ISR. In a study using a highly selective mTOR kinase inhibitor (ie, Torin2, which has less effect on calcium level in cells), more inflammatory cell adhesion (indicative of neoatherosclerosis) was observed in DES than in BMS or Torin2-eluting stents, suggesting that mTOR inhibitors play an important role in the process of neoatherosclerosis.[63]

IMAGING MODALITY FOR ASSESSMENT OF IN-STENT RESTENOSIS
Computed Tomographic Angiography

Coronary angiography (CAG) is the gold standard for the detection of ISR and R-ISR, whereas coronary computed tomographic angiography (CCTA) is also widely used in clinical practice as a noninvasive imaging modality for the detection of ISR. As compared with CAG, CCTA has been shown to have better diagnostic accuracy for ISR, both in its sensitivity (80%–90%) and negative likelihood ratio (0.1%–0.2%).[64,65] On the other hand, the limitation of CCTA is that the resolution is affected by 2 types of artifacts, blooming artifacts, due to low spatial resolution, and beam hardening artifacts, due to hard structures such as stents and calcification. These artifacts result in artificial lumen narrowing, reduced intraluminal attenuation, and overestimation of stent size.[66]

However, in recent years, CT technology has also developed significantly, and advanced imaging techniques such as dual-source CT (DSCT) and 320-row CCTA have been shown to have higher resolution, fewer artifacts, and less dependence on heart rate. In the diagnosis of ISR, DSCT and 320-row CCTA have reported higher sensitivity (92% and 91%, respectively) and specificity (91% and 95%, respectively) compared with CAG.[67] Subtraction CTA is also an effective tool for correcting artifacts due to coronary stents and calcification.[68] Subtraction CTA significantly improves the diagnostic accuracy in detecting ISR compared with conventional imaging and allows assessment of the lumen in more than 80% of patients, even for stents with diameters of 2.5 to 3 mm.[69] In addition, CT-guided FFR, which incorporates a physiologic assessment component, has seen significant progress in the past years. Recent studies have shown that it is becoming a modality that can provide comparable ischemia assessment compared to intravascular FFR.[70,71]

Intravascular Imaging

Commonly used intravascular imaging modalities include IVUS, optical coherence tomography (OCT), and near-infrared spectroscopy (NIRS). Although CAG is mainly used to assess lumen stenosis, these imaging modalities are also capable of characterizing vessel wall and plaque morphology. Intravascular imaging techniques avoid the constraints of multiple structural artifacts and improve diagnostic performance.

IVUS is a useful modality that can detect intimal hyperplasia (IH) in the assessment of ISR.[72] In the assessment of ISR in DES, CAG and IVUS parameters correlated with the rate of IH by IVUS and reliably predicted binary ISR in quantitative coronary angiography. IVUS-guided assessment of stent underexpansion, stent position, and underlying plaque morphology are potential markers for early detection of R-ISR. The evaluation of IVUS-guided stent underexpansion, stent position, and underlying plaque morphology has been envisioned as a marker for early detection of R-ISR.[73]

OCT uses near-infrared light to image and provides images with enhanced visibility of neointimal tissue. OCT provides detailed information on plaque characteristics, including lipid content, macrophage accumulation, and other calcifications. As neoatherosclerosis develops earlier in first-generation DES than in BMS and second-generation DES and is considered a cause of late ISR and late stent failure,[74–76] it is important to assess the characteristics of ISR by intravascular imaging. OCT is superior to IVUS in detecting neoatherosclerosis as IVUS has a limited ability to detect neoatherosclerosis in terms of resolution[77–79] (**Fig. 2**). Neointimal hyperplasia is characterized as a homogeneous, high-intensity layer on OCT.[80] In ISR after second-generation DES implantation, OCT has provided insight into the distinction between early (within 1 year) ISR characterized by homogeneous neointimal hyperplasia and late (after 1 year) ISR characterized by neoatherosclerosis with thin cap fibroblastoma (TCFA) and lipid-rich neointima.[76,80]

NIRS is one of the newer intravascular imaging modalities in comparison with IVUS and OCT, and the lipid core burden index (LCBI) is commonly used to quantitatively assess the size of lipid plaque. In ISR lesions, it has been reported that the minimum cap thickness of neoatherosclerosis measured by OCT correlates with maxLCBI4mm (maximum LCBI per 4 mm). Hence, NIRS can also predict the presence of neoatherosclerosis with TCFA in lipids in the stented lesion.[81]

For the use of these imaging modalities in a clinical setting, current AHA guidelines recommend that IVUS should only be used to understand the mechanism of ISR and not for routine screening objectives.[82] It is also important to understand that these imaging modalities are invasive studies, and consideration should be given to the overall indications for their use, including their cost-effectiveness in the evaluation of ISR lesions in the combination with other diagnostic modalities.

TREATMENT

Inflammation is an important factor affecting the development of ISR after stent implantation. In the past, preventing ISR and other late complications has been attempted by targeting proinflammatory pathways.[83] However, several attempts such as local nonstent or DCB-based administration of abciximab, oral sirolimus, oral corticosteroids, and paclitaxel have had limited efficacy as primary therapy.[80,84] At present, the treatment of ISR mainly involves direct interventional manipulation of the lesion. Current European guidelines recommend DES or DCB for the treatment of ISR, after consideration of intravascular imaging such as OCT[85] as an adjunctive guide.

Plain Old Balloon Angioplasty/Cutting Balloon/Scoring Balloon

Historically, plain old balloon angioplasty (POBA) has been the first device to be used for ISR therapy.[86] For underexpansion of stents, the use of noncompliant balloons capable of pressures as high as 40 atm can provide effective

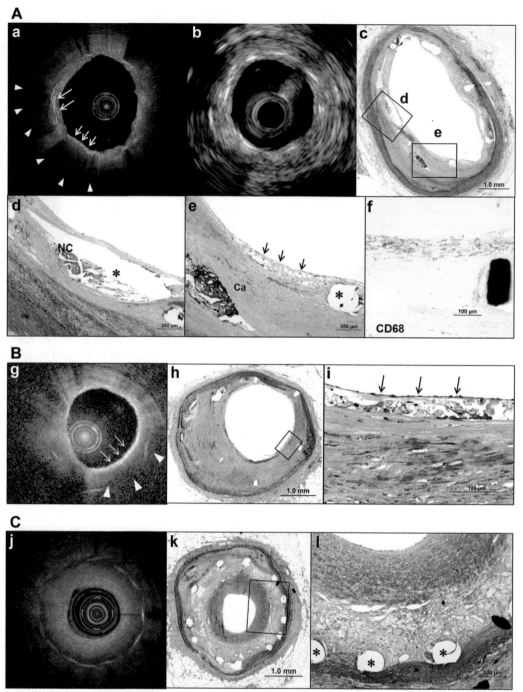

Fig. 2. Ex vivo intravascular imaging with corresponding histologic sections showing stented coronary lesions with (*A, B*) and without (*C*) neoatherosclerosis. (*a, j*) Optical coherence tomography images. (*g*) Optical frequency domain imaging image. (*b*) Intravascular ultrasound image. (*A, B*) Neoatherosclerosis characterized by foamy macrophage accumulation can be detected by optical coherence tomography/optical frequency domain imaging as a thin bright signal (*white arrows* in [a] and [g]) with a trailing shadow (ie, signal attenuation; *white arrowheads* in [a] and [g]). Linear, highly backscattering region (*yellow arrows* in [a]) with attenuation (*white arrowheads* in [a]) indicates the presence of cholesterol crystals in the necrotic core. The presence of superficial foamy macrophages (*black arrows* in [e] and [i]) was confirmed by immunostaining using anti-CD68 antibody (*f*). Note the presence of fragmented calcification behind the superficial foamy macrophages in (*e*), which cannot be detected by optical coherence tomography in (*a*). (*C*) Signal poor region without attenuation in the deeper intima as assessed by optical coherence tomography (*j*). The corresponding histologic images (*k, l*) show granulation tissue consisting of extracellular matrix and angiogenesis with varying degree of inflammatory cells. *Stent strut. (*A, C*) *Reproduced with permission from* Otsuka and colleagues.[57] (*B*) *Reproduced with permission from* Nakano and colleagues.[109]

dilation.[87] Careful attention should be given to avoid any unnecessary tissue damage due to slippage out of the stent ("watermelon seed effect"), especially when using the balloon's shorter length.[88] Scoring balloons have been introduced to reduce injury and minimize the risk of slippage on the vessel wall when inflated in ISR lesions. However, these devices alone are less effective in ISR with diffuse neointima formation and show a better result in combination with other therapeutic devices. In the ISAR-DESIRE 4 (Intracoronary Stenting and Angiographic Results) randomized trial, modification of the neointima with a scoring balloon improved the effect of DCB treatment on ISR lesions after the DES implantation.[89]

In-Stent Drug-Eluting Stent Implantation/ Drug-Coated Balloon

In a meta-analysis of treatment strategies for DES-ISR with additional DES implantation, there was a significant reduction in both TLR and target vessel revascularization compared with angioplasty alone.[90] The RIBS III trial evaluated the impact of choosing a different type of DES than the one initially implanted for ISR treatment, with favorable angiographic and clinical results at 9-month follow-up.[91] There is no definitive evidence on which type of DES should be used to treat DES ISR, and there is no consensus on whether the type of stent should be changed when implanting additional DES for DES-ISR.[80]

DCBs are devices that aim to prevent neointimal formation by delivering a highly lipophilic drug (paclitaxel) through a brief attachment from the balloon surface to the lumen of the vessel. DCBs have the advantage of avoiding additional metallic material in the treatment of ISR, and the European Society of Cardiology (ESC) guidelines recommend DCBs as a principal therapeutic option (class I, level of evidence: A).[85] However, evidence for their performance is not well established compared with that of DES reimplantation. After BMS-ISR, the incidence of TLR is lower for DCB treatment compared with POBA, while comparable to that of in-stent stenting with newer-generation DES.[92–94] Furthermore, the utility of DCBs for restenosis after DES implantation is variable, with comparable or inferior efficacy to that of newer-generation DES reimplantation for late lumen loss.[95–97] Regarding the risk of revascularization, there were also comparable outcomes for DES-ISR treated with new-generation DES and DCB.[98,99] In the DAEDALUS trial, the rates of all-cause mortality/myocardial infarction/ target lesion thrombosis at 3 years were also comparable between DES and DCB treatment.[97] In addition, DCBs are less effective in ISR lesions after repeated stenting of 3 or more layers.[100] Therefore, it is important to assess the condition of the stented lesion including the number of the metal layers when making a decision about therapeutic strategy.

Atherectomy/Debulking Device/ Brachytherapy

Both rotational atherectomy and excimer laser coronary atherectomy work to debulk the lesion and improve plaque compliance. Neither of these treatments have been shown to have enough efficacy to be regarded as a standard strategy.[101–104] In lesions with calcified neoatherosclerosis or incomplete stent expansion resistant to high-pressure balloons, these procedures have an important role as "lesion modifiers" before final DES implantation or DCB. On the other hand, brachytherapy is the temporary deposition of radioisotopes into the lesion to suppress neointimal formation. Although it showed a significant reduction in restenosis rates, there was a noted association with late recurrence.[105] Clinical results showed that ISR treatment with DES was superior to brachytherapy in the reduction of restenosis rates and the necessity for revascularization after 5 years, resulting in its rare use in the treatment of ISR currently.[106,107] However, brachytherapy still has a role in the treatment of DES-ISR, especially in recurrent lesions with multiple stent layers, where it is an option to avoid additional metal layers.[80]

SUMMARY

Here we summarized the mechanisms of ISR that have been elucidated so far, the evaluation of ISR using different imaging modalities, and the currently available primary treatment options. Even with newer-generation DES, ISR remains the Achilles heel of PCI, and it is essential to consider the mechanism of ISR and histologic findings in the selection of therapeutic options, while technical perspectives will require further improvement in stent performance. Given the mechanism of ISR, the ideal DES should consist of a platform that strikes a balance between reducing restenosis and minimizing delayed vessel healing. The performance of DES materials, such as strut thickness, drugs, polymers, and deliverability, is expected to improve in the future, following the history of improvements in DES initiated with the first generation.

CLINICS CARE POINTS

- Histologic characteristics of BMS-ISR are diffuse patterns with predominant VSMC and less ECM, whereas DES-ISR has a focal pattern with rich extracellular matrix deposition and hypocellularity in neointima.

- Hypersensitivity and local inflammation after DES implantation, as well as delayed healing, are major factors in neointimal formation causing ISR.

- Neoatherosclerosis is one of the hallmarks of ISR and can be observed in both BMS and DES. The progression of neoatherosclerosis is earlier in DES than in BMS.

- Angiography is the gold standard for morphologic evaluation of ISR, whereas intravascular imaging, such as IVUS and OCT, is useful for tissue assessments including neoatherosclerosis and can be used to guide therapeutic options.

- DCB and repeat DES implantation is the standard treatment option for ISR currently, but the evidence for the efficacy of DCB is not necessarily superior to that of DES, and the choice should be based on patient background and lesion morphology.

DISCLOSURE

CVPath Institute received Grant/Research/Clinical Trial Support from NIH-HL141425, Leducq Foundation Grant, 4C Medical, 4Tech, Abbott Vascular, Ablative Solutions, Absorption Systems, Advanced NanoTherapies, Aerwave Medical, Alivas, Amgen, Asahi Medical, Aurios Medical, Avantec Vascular, BD, Biosensors, Biotronik, Biotyx Medical, Bolt Medical, Boston Scientific, Canon USA, Cardiac Implants, Cardiawave, Cardio-Mech, Cardionomic, Celonova, Cerus EndoVascular, Chansu Vascular Technologies, Childrens National Medical Center, Concept Medical, Cook Medical, Cooper Health, Cormaze Technologies GmbH, CRL/AccelLab, Croivalve, CSI, Dexcom, Edwards Lifesciences, Elucid Bioimaging, Emboline, Endotronix, Envision, Filterlex, Imperative Care, Innovalve, Innovative Cardiovascular Solutions, Intact Vascular, Interface Biolgics, Intershunt Technologies, Invatin Technologies, Lahav CRO, Limflow, L&J Biosciences, Lutonix, Lyra Therapeutics, Mayo Clinic, Maywell, MD Start, MedAlliance, Medanex, Medtronic, Mercator, Microport, Microvention, Neovasc, Nephronyx, Nova Vascular, Nyra Medical, Occultech, Olympus, Ohio Health, OrbusNeich, Ossio, Phenox, Pi-Cardia, Polares Medical, Polyvascular, Profusa, ProKidney LLC, Protembis, Pulse Biosciences, Qool Therapeutics, Recombinetics, Recor Medical, Regencor, Renata Medical, Restore Medical, Ripple Therapeutics, Rush University, Sanofi, Shockwave, Sahajan and Medical Technologies, Sound-Pipe, Spartan Micro, Spectrawave, Surmodics, Terumo Corporation, The Jacobs Institute, Transmural Systems, Transverse Medical, TruLeaf Medical, UCSF, UPMC, Vascudyne, Vesper, Vetex Medical, Whiteswell, WL Gore, and Xeltis. A.V. Finn received consultant fees/honoraria from Abbott Vascular, Amgen, Biosensors, Boston Scientific, Celonova, Cook Medical, CSI, Lutonix Bard, Sinomed, and Terumo Corporation. R. Virmani is a consultant of Abbott Vascular, Boston Scientific, Celonova, OrbusNeich Medical, Terumo Corporation, W. L. Gore, Edwards Lifesciences, Cook Medical, CSI, ReCor Medical, SinoMedical Sciences Technology, Surmodics, Bard BD and is a Scientific Advisory Board Member of Medtronic and Xeltis. Kenji Kawai has no other relevant affiliations or financial involvement with any organization or entity with a financial interest in or financial conflict with the subject matter or materials discussed.

REFERENCES

1. Cutlip DE, Chhabra AG, Baim DS, et al. Beyond restenosis: five-year clinical outcomes from second-generation coronary stent trials. Circulation 2004;110:1226–30.

2. Waldo SW, O'Donnell CI, Prouse A, et al. Incidence, procedural management, and clinical outcomes of coronary in-stent restenosis: Insights from the National VA CART Program. Catheter Cardiovasc Interv 2018;91:425–33.

3. Moussa ID, Mohananey D, Saucedo J, et al. Trends and outcomes of restenosis after coronary stent implantation in the united states. J Am Coll Cardiol 2020;76:1521–31.

4. Mehran R, Dangas G, Abizaid AS, et al. Angiographic patterns of in-stent restenosis: classification and implications for long-term outcome. Circulation 1999;100:1872–8.

5. Alfonso F, Byrne RA, Rivero F, et al. Current treatment of in-stent restenosis. J Am Coll Cardiol 2014;63:2659–73.

6. Alfonso F, Cequier A, Angel J, et al. Value of the American college of cardiology/american heart association angiographic classification of coronary lesion morphology in patients with in-stent restenosis. insights from the restenosis intra-stent balloon angioplasty versus elective Stenting (RIBS) randomized trial. Am Heart J 2006;151:681 e1–9.

7. Cutlip DE, Windecker S, Mehran R, et al. Clinical end points in coronary stent trials: a case for standardized definitions. Circulation 2007;115:2344–51.

8. Dangas GD, Claessen BE, Caixeta A, et al. In-stent restenosis in the drug-eluting stent era. J Am Coll Cardiol 2010;56:1897–907.

9. Abizaid AS, Mintz GS, Mehran R, et al. Long-term follow-up after percutaneous transluminal coronary angioplasty was not performed based on intravascular ultrasound findings: importance of lumen dimensions. Circulation 1999;100:256–61.

10. Jasti V, Ivan E, Yalamanchili V, et al. Correlations between fractional flow reserve and intravascular ultrasound in patients with an ambiguous left main coronary artery stenosis. Circulation 2004; 110:2831–6.

11. Doi H, Maehara A, Mintz GS, et al. Impact of in-stent minimal lumen area at 9 months poststent implantation on 3-year target lesion revascularization-free survival: a serial intravascular ultrasound analysis from the TAXUS IV, V, and VI trials. Circ Cardiovasc Interv 2008;1:111–8.

12. Kawamoto H, Ruparelia N, Latib A, et al. Drug-coated balloons versus second-generation drug-eluting stents for the management of recurrent multimetal-layered in-stent restenosis. JACC Cardiovasc Interv 2015;8:1586–94.

13. Waksman R, Iantorno M. Refractory in-stent restenosis: improving outcomes by standardizing our approach. Curr Cardiol Rep 2018;20:140.

14. Stettler C, Wandel S, Allemann S, et al. Outcomes associated with drug-eluting and bare-metal stents: a collaborative network meta-analysis. Lancet 2007;370:937–48.

15. Byrne RA, Sarafoff N, Kastrati A, et al. Drug-eluting stents in percutaneous coronary intervention: a benefit-risk assessment. Drug Saf 2009;32: 749–70.

16. Moses JW, Leon MB, Popma JJ, et al. Sirolimus-eluting stents versus standard stents in patients with stenosis in a native coronary artery. N Engl J Med 2003;349:1315–23.

17. Serruys PW, Silber S, Garg S, et al. Comparison of zotarolimus-eluting and everolimus-eluting coronary stents. N Engl J Med 2010;363:136–46.

18. Kozuma K, Kimura T, Kadota K, et al. Angiographic findings of everolimus-eluting as compared to sirolimus-eluting stents: angiographic sub-study from the Randomized Evaluation of Sirolimus-eluting versus Everolimus-eluting stent Trial (RESET). Cardiovasc Interv Ther 2013;28:344–51.

19. Aoki J, Kozuma K, Awata M, et al. Three-year clinical outcomes of everolimus-eluting stents from the post-marketing surveillance study of cobalt-chromium everolimus-eluting stent (XIENCE V/PROMUS) in Japan. Circ J 2016;80:906–12.

20. Piccolo R, Stefanini GG, Franzone A, et al. Safety and efficacy of resolute zotarolimus-eluting stents compared with everolimus-eluting stents: a meta-analysis. Circ Cardiovasc Interv 2015;8:e002223.

21. Aoki J, Tanabe K. Mechanisms of drug-eluting stent restenosis. Cardiovasc Interv Ther 2021;36:23–9.

22. Theodoropoulos K, Mennuni MG, Dangas GD, et al. Resistant in-stent restenosis in the drug eluting stent era. Catheter Cardiovasc Interv 2016;88:777–85.

23. Zahn R, Hamm CW, Schneider S, et al. Incidence and predictors of target vessel revascularization and clinical event rates of the sirolimus-eluting coronary stent (results from the prospective multi-center German Cypher Stent Registry). Am J Cardiol 2005;95:1302–8.

24. Zahn R, Hamm CW, Schneider S, et al. Coronary stenting with the sirolimus-eluting stent in clinical practice: final results from the prospective multi-center German Cypher Stent Registry. J Interv Cardiol 2010;23:18–25.

25. Kastrati A, Dibra A, Mehilli J, et al. Predictive factors of restenosis after coronary implantation of sirolimus- or paclitaxel-eluting stents. Circulation 2006;113:2293–300.

26. Sakamoto A, Sato Y, Kawakami R, et al. Risk prediction of in-stent restenosis among patients with coronary drug-eluting stents: current clinical approaches and challenges. Expert Rev Cardiovasc Ther 2021;19:801–16.

27. Doi H, Maehara A, Mintz GS, et al. Impact of post-intervention minimal stent area on 9-month follow-up patency of paclitaxel-eluting stents: an integrated intravascular ultrasound analysis from the TAXUS IV, V, and VI and TAXUS ATLAS work-horse, long lesion, and direct stent trials. JACC Cardiovasc Interv 2009;2:1269–75.

28. Morino Y, Honda Y, Okura H, et al. An optimal diagnostic threshold for minimal stent area to predict target lesion revascularization following stent implantation in native coronary lesions. Am J Cardiol 2001;88:301–3.

29. Sonoda S, Morino Y, Ako J, et al. Impact of final stent dimensions on long-term results following sirolimus-eluting stent implantation: serial intravascular ultrasound analysis from the sirius trial. J Am Coll Cardiol 2004;43:1959–63.

30. Song HG, Kang SJ, Ahn JM, et al. Intravascular ultrasound assessment of optimal stent area to prevent in-stent restenosis after zotarolimus-, everolimus-, and sirolimus-eluting stent implantation. Catheter Cardiovasc Interv 2014;83:873–8.

31. Pepe M, Napoli G, Carulli E, et al. Autoimmune diseases in patients undergoing percutaneous coronary intervention: A risk factor for in-stent restenosis? Atherosclerosis 2021;333:24–31.

32. Danenberg HD, Welt FG, Walker M 3rd, et al. Systemic inflammation induced by lipopolysaccha-ride increases neointimal formation after balloon and stent injury in rabbits. Circulation 2002;105: 2917–22.

33. Shah PK. Inflammation, neointimal hyperplasia, and restenosis: as the leukocytes roll, the arteries thicken. Circulation 2003;107:2175–7.

34. Serrano MC, Vavra AK, Jen M, et al. Poly(diol-co-citrate)s as novel elastomeric perivascular wraps for the reduction of neointimal hyperplasia. Macromol Biosci 2011;11:700–9.

35. Kim MS, Dean LS. In-stent restenosis. Cardiovasc Ther 2011;29:190–8.

36. Mori H, Finn AV, Atkinson JB, et al. Calcified nodule: an early and late cause of in-stent failure. JACC Cardiovasc Interv 2016;9:e125–6.

37. Moses JW, Usui E, Maehara A. Recognition of recurrent stent failure due to calcified nodule: between a rock and a hard place. JACC Case Rep 2020;2:1879–81.

38. Kawai K, Akahori H, Imanaka T, et al. Coronary restenosis of in-stent protruding bump with rapid progression: Optical frequency domain imaging and angioscopic observation. J Cardiol Cases 2018;19(1):12–4.

39. Schwartz RS, Huber KC, Murphy JG, et al. Restenosis and the proportional neointimal response to coronary artery injury: results in a porcine model. J Am Coll Cardiol 1992;19:267–74.

40. Farb A, Weber DK, Kolodgie FD, et al. Morphological predictors of restenosis after coronary stenting in humans. Circulation 2002;105:2974–80.

41. Welt FG, Rogers C. Inflammation and restenosis in the stent era. Arterioscler Thromb Vasc Biol 2002;22:1769–76.

42. Chung IM, Gold HK, Schwartz SM, et al. Enhanced extracellular matrix accumulation in restenosis of coronary arteries after stent deployment. J Am Coll Cardiol 2002;40:2072–81.

43. Schwartz RS, Holmes DR Jr, Topol EJ. The restenosis paradigm revisited: an alternative proposal for cellular mechanisms. J Am Coll Cardiol 1992; 20:1284–93.

44. Rosenthal N, Costa MA. Unravelling the endovascular microenvironment by optical coherence tomography. Eur Heart J 2010;31:139–42.

45. Pleva L, Kukla P, Hlinomaz O. Treatment of coronary in-stent restenosis: a systematic review. J Geriatr Cardiol 2018;15:173–84.

46. Lee SY, Hong MK, Jang Y. Formation and transformation of neointima after drug-eluting stent implantation: insights from optical coherence tomographic studies. Korean Circ J 2017;47: 823–32.

47. Nakamura D, Yasumura K, Nakamura H, et al. Different neoatherosclerosis patterns in drug-eluting- and bare-metal stent restenosis - optical coherence tomography study. Circ J 2019;83: 313–9.

48. Nakano M, Otsuka F, Yahagi K, et al. Human autopsy study of drug-eluting stents restenosis: histomorphological predictors and neointimal characteristics. Eur Heart J 2013;34:3304–13.

49. Claessen BE, Stone GW, Mehran R, et al. Relationship between biomarkers and subsequent clinical and angiographic restenosis after paclitaxel-eluting stents for treatment of STEMI: a HORIZONS-AMI substudy. J Thromb Thrombolysis 2012;34:165–79.

50. Katsaros KM, Kastl SP, Zorn G, et al. Increased restenosis rate after implantation of drug-eluting stents in patients with elevated serum activity of matrix metalloproteinase-2 and -9. JACC Cardiovasc Interv 2010;3:90–7.

51. Park DW, Hong MK, Mintz GS, et al. Two-year follow-up of the quantitative angiographic and volumetric intravascular ultrasound analysis after nonpolymeric paclitaxel-eluting stent implantation: late "catch-up" phenomenon from ASPECT Study. J Am Coll Cardiol 2006;48:2432–9.

52. Kang SJ, Park DW, Mintz GS, et al. Long-term vascular changes after drug-eluting stent implantation assessed by serial volumetric intravascular ultrasound analysis. Am J Cardiol 2010;105:1402–8.

53. Byrne RA, Joner M, Tada T, et al. Restenosis in bare metal and drug-eluting stents: distinct mechanistic insights from histopathology and optical intravascular imaging. Minerva Cardioangiol 2012;60:473–89.

54. Nakazawa G, Otsuka F, Nakano M, et al. The pathology of neoatherosclerosis in human coronary implants bare-metal and drug-eluting stents. J Am Coll Cardiol 2011;57:1314–22.

55. Glover C, Ma X, Chen YX, et al. Human in-stent restenosis tissue obtained by means of coronary atherectomy consists of an abundant proteoglycan matrix with a paucity of cell proliferation. Am Heart J 2002;144:702–9.

56. Park SJ, Kang SJ, Virmani R, et al. In-stent neoatherosclerosis: a final common pathway of late stent failure. J Am Coll Cardiol 2012;59:2051–7.

57. Otsuka F, Byrne RA, Yahagi K, et al. Neoatherosclerosis: overview of histopathologic findings and implications for intravascular imaging assessment. Eur Heart J 2015;36:2147–59.

58. Joner M, Nakazawa G, Finn AV, et al. Endothelial cell recovery between comparator polymer-based drug-eluting stents. J Am Coll Cardiol 2008;52: 333–42.

59. Nakazawa G, Nakano M, Otsuka F, et al. Evaluation of polymer-based comparator drug-eluting stents using a rabbit model of iliac artery atherosclerosis. Circ Cardiovasc Interv 2011;4:38–46.

60. Otsuka F, Finn AV, Yazdani SK, et al. The importance of the endothelium in atherothrombosis and coronary stenting. Nat Rev Cardiol 2012;9: 439–53.

61. Otsuka F, Pacheco E, Perkins LE, et al. Long-term safety of an everolimus-eluting bioresorbable vascular scaffold and the cobalt-chromium XIENCE V stent in a porcine coronary artery model. Circ Cardiovasc Interv 2014;7:330–42.

62. Habib A, Karmali V, Polavarapu R, et al. Sirolimus-FKBP12.6 impairs endothelial barrier function through protein kinase C-α activation and disruption of the p120-vascular endothelial cadherin interaction. Arterioscler Thromb Vasc Biol 2013; 33:2425–31.

63. Harari E, Guo L, Smith SL, et al. Direct targeting of the mTOR (Mammalian Target of Rapamycin) kinase improves endothelial permeability in drug-eluting stents-brief report. Arterioscler Thromb Vasc Biol 2018;38:2217–24.

64. Carrabba N, Schuijf JD, de Graaf FR, et al. Diagnostic accuracy of 64-slice computed tomography coronary angiography for the detection of in-stent restenosis: a meta-analysis. J Nucl Cardiol 2010; 17:470–8.

65. Hamon M, Champ-Rigot L, Morello R, et al. Diagnostic accuracy of in-stent coronary restenosis detection with multislice spiral computed tomography: a meta-analysis. Eur Radiol 2008;18:217–25.

66. de Graaf FR, Schuijf JD, van Velzen JE, et al. Diagnostic accuracy of 320-row multidetector computed tomography coronary angiography to noninvasively assess in-stent restenosis. Invest Radiol 2010;45:331–40.

67. Liu HF, Wang M, Xu YS, et al. Diagnostic accuracy of dual-source and 320-row computed tomography angiography in detecting coronary in-stent restenosis: a systematic review and meta-analysis. Acta Radiol 2019;60:149–59.

68. Yoshihara S, Kamiya M, Yaegashi T, et al. Subtraction coronary CT angiography clarifies in-stent restenosis of a three-layer stent segment. Acta Cardiol 2017;72:226–7.

69. Amanuma M, Kondo T, Sano T, et al. Assessment of coronary in-stent restenosis: value of subtraction coronary computed tomography angiography. Int J Cardiovasc Imaging 2016;32:661–70.

70. Tang CX, Wang YN, Zhou F, et al. Diagnostic performance of fractional flow reserve derived from coronary CT angiography for detection of lesion-specific ischemia: A multi-center study and meta-analysis. Eur J Radiol 2019;116:90–7.

71. Ko BS, Linde JJ, Ihdayhid AR, et al. Non-invasive CT-derived fractional flow reserve and static rest and stress CT myocardial perfusion imaging for detection of haemodynamically significant coronary stenosis. Int J Cardiovasc Imaging 2019;35: 2103–12.

72. Escolar E, Mintz GS, Popma J, et al. Meta-analysis of angiographic versus intravascular ultrasound parameters of drug-eluting stent efficacy (from TAXUS IV, V, and VI). Am J Cardiol 2007;100: 621–6.

73. Spanos V, Stankovic G, Tobis J, et al. The challenge of in-stent restenosis: insights from intravascular ultrasound. Eur Heart J 2003;24:138–50.

74. Habara M, Terashima M, Nasu K, et al. Morphological differences of tissue characteristics between early, late, and very late restenosis lesions after first generation drug-eluting stent implantation: an optical coherence tomography study. Eur Heart J Cardiovasc Imaging 2013;14:276–84.

75. Kajiya T, Yamaguchi H, Takaoka J, et al. In-stent restenosis assessed with frequency domain optical coherence tomography shows smooth coronary arterial healing process in second-generation drug-eluting stents. Singapore Med J 2019;60: 48–51.

76. Jinnouchi H, Kuramitsu S, Shinozaki T, et al. Difference of tissue characteristics between early and late restenosis after second-generation drug-eluting stents implantation - an optical coherence tomography study. Circ J 2017;81:450–7.

77. Ali ZA, Roleder T, Narula J, et al. Increased thin-cap neoatheroma and periprocedural myocardial infarction in drug-eluting stent restenosis: multi-modality intravascular imaging of drug-eluting and bare-metal stents. Circ Cardiovasc Interv 2013;6:507–17.

78. Fujii K, Kawakami R, Hirota S. Histopathological validation of optical coherence tomography findings of the coronary arteries. J Cardiol 2018;72:179–85.

79. Suzuki Y, Ikeno F, Koizumi T, et al. In vivo comparison between optical coherence tomography and intravascular ultrasound for detecting small degrees of in-stent neointima after stent implantation. JACC Cardiovasc Interv 2008;1:168–73.

80. Shlofmitz E, Iantorno M, Waksman R. Restenosis of Drug-Eluting Stents: A New Classification System Based on Disease Mechanism to Guide Treatment and State-of-the-Art Review. Circ Cardiovasc Interv 2019;12:e007023.

81. Roleder T, Karimi Galoughahi K, Chin CY, et al. Utility of near-infrared spectroscopy for detection of thin-cap neoatherosclerosis. Eur Heart J Cardiovasc Imaging 2017;18:663–9.

82. Levine GN, Bates ER, Blankenship JC, et al. ACCF/AHA/SCAI guideline for percutaneous coronary intervention: a report of the american college of cardiology foundation/american heart association task force on practice guidelines and the society for cardiovascular angiography and interventions. Circulation 2011;124:e574–651.

83. Borovac JA, D'Amario D, Vergallo R, et al. Neoatherosclerosis after drug-eluting stent implantation: a novel clinical and therapeutic challenge. Eur Heart J Cardiovasc Pharmacother 2019;5: 105–16.

84. Cassese S, De Luca G, Ribichini F, et al. ORAl iMmunosuppressive therapy to prevent in-Stent rEstenosiS (RAMSES) cooperation: a patient-level meta-analysis of randomized trials. Atherosclerosis 2014;237:410–7.

85. Neumann FJ, Sousa-Uva M, Ahlsson A, et al. ESC/EACTS Guidelines on myocardial revascularization. Eur Heart J 2019;40:87–165.

86. Kastrati A, Mehilli J, von Beckerath N, et al. Sirolimus-eluting stent or paclitaxel-eluting stent vs balloon angioplasty for prevention of recurrences in patients with coronary in-stent restenosis: a randomized controlled trial. JAMA 2005;293:165–71.

87. Felekos I, Karamasis GV, Pavlidis AN. When everything else fails: High-pressure balloon for undilatable lesions. Cardiovasc Revasc Med 2018;19:306–13.

88. Alfonso F, Pérez-Vizcayno MJ, Gómez-Recio M, et al. Implications of the "watermelon seeding" phenomenon during coronary interventions for in-stent restenosis. Catheter Cardiovasc Interv 2005;66:521–7.

89. Colleran R, Joner M, Kufner S, et al. Comparative efficacy of two paclitaxel-coated balloons with different excipient coatings in patients with coronary in-stent restenosis: a pooled analysis of the intracoronary stenting and angiographic results: optimizing treatment of drug eluting stent in-stent restenosis 3 and 4 (ISAR-DESIRE 3 and ISAR-DESIRE 4) trials. Int J Cardiol 2018;252:57–62.

90. Goel SS, Dilip Gajulapalli R, Athappan G, et al. Management of drug eluting stent in-stent restenosis: A systematic review and meta-analysis. Catheter Cardiovasc Interv 2016;87:1080–91.

91. Alfonso F, Pérez-Vizcayno MJ, Dutary J, et al. Implantation of a drug-eluting stent with a different drug (switch strategy) in patients with drug-eluting stent restenosis. Results from a prospective multicenter study (RIBS III [restenosis intra-stent: balloon angioplasty versus drug-eluting stent]). JACC Cardiovasc Interv 2012;5:728–37.

92. Alfonso F, Pérez-Vizcayno MJ, Cárdenas A, et al. A randomized comparison of drug-eluting balloon versus everolimus-eluting stent in patients with bare-metal stent-in-stent restenosis: the RIBS V clinical trial (restenosis intra-stent of bare metal stents: paclitaxel-eluting balloon vs. everolimus-eluting stent). J Am Coll Cardiol 2014;63:1378–86.

93. Pleva L, Kukla P, Kusnierova P, et al. Comparison of the Efficacy of Paclitaxel-Eluting Balloon Catheters and Everolimus-Eluting Stents in the Treatment of Coronary In-Stent Restenosis: The Treatment of In-Stent Restenosis Study. Circ Cardiovasc Interv 2016;9:e003316.

94. Lee JM, Park J, Kang J, et al. Comparison among drug-eluting balloon, drug-eluting stent, and plain balloon angioplasty for the treatment of in-stent restenosis: a network meta-analysis of 11 randomized, controlled trials. JACC Cardiovasc Interv 2015;8:382–94.

95. Cai JZ, Zhu YX, Wang XY, et al. Comparison of new-generation drug-eluting stents versus drug-coated balloon for in-stent restenosis: a meta-analysis of randomised controlled trials. BMJ Open 2018;8:e017231.

96. Giacoppo D, Alfonso F, Xu B, et al. Drug-coated balloon angioplasty versus drug-eluting stent implantation in patients with coronary stent restenosis. J Am Coll Cardiol 2020;75:2664–78.

97. Giacoppo D, Alfonso F, Xu B, et al. Paclitaxel-coated balloon angioplasty vs. drug-eluting stenting for the treatment of coronary in-stent restenosis: a comprehensive, collaborative, individual patient data meta-analysis of 10 randomized clinical trials (DAEDALUS study). Eur Heart J 2020;41:3715–28.

98. Siontis GC, Stefanini GG, Mavridis D, et al. Percutaneous coronary interventional strategies for treatment of in-stent restenosis: a network meta-analysis. Lancet 2015;386:655–64.

99. Giacoppo D, Gargiulo G, Aruta P, et al. Treatment strategies for coronary in-stent restenosis: systematic review and hierarchical Bayesian network meta-analysis of 24 randomised trials and 4880 patients. BMJ 2015;351:h5392.

100. Yabushita H, Kawamoto H, Fujino Y, et al. Clinical outcomes of drug-eluting balloon for in-stent restenosis based on the number of metallic layers. Circ Cardiovasc Interv 2018;11:e005935.

101. vom Dahl J, Dietz U, Haager PK, et al. Rotational atherectomy does not reduce recurrent in-stent restenosis: results of the angioplasty versus rotational atherectomy for treatment of diffuse in-stent restenosis trial (ARTIST). Circulation 2002;105:583–8.

102. Sharma SK, Kini A, Mehran R, et al. Randomized trial of rotational atherectomy versus balloon angioplasty for diffuse in-stent restenosis (ROSTER). Am Heart J 2004;147:16–22.

103. Mehran R, Mintz GS, Satler LF, et al. Treatment of in-stent restenosis with excimer laser coronary angioplasty: mechanisms and results compared with PTCA alone. Circulation 1997;96:2183–9.

104. Radke PW, Kaiser A, Frost C, et al. Outcome after treatment of coronary in-stent restenosis; results from a systematic review using meta-analysis techniques. Eur Heart J 2003;24:266–73.

105. Leon MB, Teirstein PS, Moses JW, et al. Localized intracoronary gamma-radiation therapy to inhibit the recurrence of restenosis after stenting. N Engl J Med 2001;344:250–6.

106. Holmes DR Jr, Teirstein P, Satler L, et al. Sirolimus-eluting stents vs vascular brachytherapy

for in-stent restenosis within bare-metal stents: the SISR randomized trial. JAMA 2006;295: 1264–73.

107. Stone GW, Ellis SG, O'Shaughnessy CD, et al. Paclitaxel-eluting stents vs vascular brachytherapy for in-stent restenosis within bare-metal stents: the TAXUS V ISR randomized trial. JAMA 2006; 295:1253–63.

108. Otsuka F, Vorpahl M, Nakano M, et al. Pathology of second-generation everolimus-eluting stents versus first-generation sirolimus- and paclitaxel-eluting stents in humans. Circulation 2014;129:211–23.

109. Nakano M, Vorpahl M, Otsuka F, et al. Ex vivo assessment of vascular response to coronary stents by optical frequency domain imaging. JACC Cardiovasc Imaging 2012;5:71–82.

Management of Coronary Complications

David M. Tehrani, MD, MS[a],*, Arnold H. Seto, MD, MPA, FSCAI[b]

KEYWORDS

- Coronary dissection • Coronary perforation • Abrupt vessel closure • No-reflow
- Device embolization

KEY POINTS

- With the advancement in tools to allow for more complex percutaneous coronary intervention (PCI), the possibility of procedural complication has also grown.
- In-depth knowledge of possible coronary complications, allow operators to plan for complications and prevent them from occurring.
- Rapid identification and management of coronary complications will lead to improved outcomes.

INTRODUCTION

Percutaneous coronary intervention (PCI) has made significant advancements in the treatment of obstructive coronary artery disease over the past 5 decades. Advancements in antiplatelet therapy, anticoagulation strategies, stent delivery systems, atherectomy devices, balloons, embolic protection devices, and stent design have helped make PCI an increasingly safe procedure. However, major periprocedural complications can occur with PCI, with a risk of death and periprocedural myocardial infarction (MI) of 0.1%.[1] The focus of this article will be on the prevention, identification, and treatment of coronary complications including perforation, abrupt vessel closure, device embolization (stent and wire), and rotational atherectomy burr entrapment during PCI.

GENERAL RISK OF PERCUTANEOUS CORONARY INTERVENTION

Complication rates after PCI vary widely based on patient and procedural factors. Compared with diagnostic studies the rate of complications is much higher. Patients undergoing PCI are at high risk for long-term adverse outcomes with approximately20% risk of repeat revascularization within the first year following PCI, as well as MI or cerebrovascular accident (CVA).[2,3] Here we focus on periprocedural complications of PCI.

Periprocedural Myocardial Infarction

The general risk of periprocedural (Type 4a) MI is challenging to fully describe, as various definitions have evolved with the availability of increasingly sensitive troponin assays.[2] There is no universal consensus on the cut-offs of cardiac troponin (cTn) or high-sensitivity cardiac troponin (hs-cTn). Rather, the distinction should be made based on an injury that creates a flow-limiting state.[2] In general the criteria for a cardiac procedural MI is arbitrarily defined as an increase of cTn values (>99th percentile of the upper reference limit (URL)) in patients with normal baseline cTn value or a increase in cTn values >20% of those with baseline above the 99th percentile URL but is stable or falling.[2] For MI associated with PCI (type 4a MI), the definition requires an elevation of cTn values >5 times the 99th percentile URL in patients with normal baseline values or, in patients with

[a] University of California Los Angeles, 650 Charles East Young Drive South, A20237 CHS, Los Angeles, CA 90095, USA; [b] Long Beach Veterans Administration Medical Center, 5901 East 7th Street 111C, Long Beach, CA 90822, USA
* Corresponding author.
E-mail address: david.m.tehrani@gmail.com

Intervent Cardiol Clin 11 (2022) 445–453
https://doi.org/10.1016/j.iccl.2022.06.002
2211-7458/22/© 2022 Elsevier Inc. All rights reserved.

elevated preprocedure cTn in whom the cTn levels are stable (<20% variation) or falling, the preprocedure cTn must rise greater than 20% to absolute value >5 times the 99th percentile URL.[2] Critically, patients must also demonstrate signs or symptoms suggestive of myocardial ischemia such as electrocardiographic changes, imaging evidence of impaired flow, or procedure-related complications. This should be placed in the context of a large number of patients, ~20 to 40% in those with stable coronary artery disease and ~40–50% in those presenting with MI, that has abnormal values of cTn after PCI without such supportive signs.[3] Of note, a hs-cTn definition has not been established for type 4a MI.

The temporal trends for post-PCI CVA show an increasing incidence, based on analysis from the national inpatient sample from 2003 to 2016.[4] In general, following PCI the risk of CVA increased from 0.6% to about 1% for STEMI, 0.5% to 0.6% for NSTEMI, and 0.3% to 0.7% for unstable angina or stable ischemic disease during the study period. The risk factors associated with increased ischemic stroke post-PCI included those with carotid disease, cardiogenic shock, atrial fibrillation, older age, and low to intermediate-volume PCI centers.

With the improvement in the advancement in all facets of PCI, the need for emergency coronary artery bypass grafting (CABG) has decreased. Data from the American College of Cardiology National Cardiovascular Data Registry (NCDR) showed that the aggregate incidence of emergency CABG is low at 0.4% with the mortality of approximately 13% when emergency CABG was necessary.[5]

Short-term mortality immediately due to PCI is highly variable due to the patient's comorbidities, acuity of presentation, and PCI complexity. Older data from the NCDR between 1998 and 2000 indicated that PCI mortality averaged 1.4%.[6] Similarly, NCDR data from more than 18,000 procedures performed between 2004 and 2006 showed that overall post-PCI in-hospital morality was 1.27%, ranging from 0.65% in elective PCI to 4.81% in patients with STEMI.[7] In-hospital mortality was driven primarily by pre-existing patient's comorbidities and markers of clinical instability, while angiographic complexity added only modest predictive value.[7] Most recently, data from 700,000 PCIs performed between July 2018 and June 2019, showed that procedural urgency and cardiovascular instability were the greatest predictors of in-hospital mortality with a median hospital risk-standardized rate of 1.9% among those who

underwent PCI.[8] This shows that despite tremendous advances in PCI and medical therapy, peri-procedural mortality remains a significant concern but is driven primarily by clinical presentation. Nonetheless, when complications occur, they can be deadly, and preparation for the eventual complication can be lifesaving.

COMPLICATIONS AND MANAGEMENT OF PERCUTANEOUS CORONARY INTERVENTIONS

Coronary Perforation

Coronary perforation has an estimated incidence of approximately 0.5% and is associated with a 13-fold increase in in-hospital mortality.[9,10] It is most commonly caused by distal wire migration, followed by angioplasty balloon rupture, stent oversizing, and high-pressure postdilation. Factors associated with perforation include atherectomy devices, interventions on chronic total occlusions, increased age, female sex, and prior CABG.[10–12] Perforations can be classified according to location, which can have important implications regarding management. The 3 main perforation locations are main vessel perforations, distal artery wire perforations, and collateral vessel perforation in either a septal or an epicardial collateral.[13] Additionally, the Ellis calcification for coronary artery perforation was proposed in 1994 to grade the severity of the perforation:

- Grade I: Extraluminal crater extending outside the lumen without extravasation or linear staining angiographically suggestive of a dissection.
- Grade II: Pericardial or myocardial blushing without a greater than or equal to 1 mm diameter exit hole.
- Grade III: Frank streaming of contrast through a greater than or equal to 1 mm diameter exit hole, including perforation into an anatomic cavity such as the coronary sinus or the right ventricle.

The deadliest outcome of a coronary perforation is that of a frank rupture leading to rapid filling of the pericardial space resulting in cardiac tamponade as seen in grade III coronary perforation.

Focused technique and planning are the key to the prevention of coronary artery perforation. Avoiding distal wire migration, especially when using a hydrophilic wire, is very important with multiple passes with equipment. Diligence with final angiography is also important, as small, distal micro-perforations maybe missed leading to complications in the postprocedure timeframe. The use of intracoronary imaging can help avoid overly aggressive balloon and stent sizing.

While Ellis grade I perforations typically resolve with reversal of anticoagulation and prolonged balloon inflation, more severe perforations are more likely to persist. The focus of the management of a coronary perforation is on that of a grade III perforation and depends on severity, anatomic location, and hemodynamic compromise. After a coronary perforation is confirmed angiographically, immediate proximal balloon inflation is the critical first step to prevent continued extravasation into the pericardium. A compliant balloon should be inflated at the lowest possible pressure to promote hemostasis as confirmed by contrast injection at regular intervals. Inflation is oftentimes in the timeframe of minutes (5–10 minutes) as additional equipment is collected, secondary arterial access is obtained, and assistance is recruited. However, this may lead to ischemia of the myocardial territory fed by the perforated vessel, resulting in further hemodynamic or electrical instability. If ischemia is severe, prompt the implantation of a covered stent is in order.

Anticoagulation stoppage and reversal should be considered. Depending on the anatomy and the size of the perforated vessel, usually distal artery wire perforations and collateral vessel perforations, the use of subcutaneous fat (from the patient), the use of thrombin, or occlusive coils or beads can be used.[14–16] Small vessel perforations can often be resolved with embolization or prolonged balloon inflation, such that the risk of equipment thrombosis with reversal can be avoided (Fig. 1). Main vessel perforations (Fig. 2) require reversal with protamine sulfate (recommended dose of 1 mg IV for each 100 units of unfractionated heparin given) administered to achieve an activated clotting time of less than 150 seconds if heparin is the agent of use during PCI.[17] If bivalirudin is the agent of use during PCI, reversal can be attempted with the use of a recombinant activated factor VII, which has been used at a dose of 90 μg/kg IV. Fresh frozen plasma may also be considered for partial reversal of bivalirudin anticoagulation.[18] The relatively short half-life of bivalirudin is of benefit should bleeding occur.

Once a balloon is occlusive and a decision is made on anticoagulation reversal, aggressive supportive care with intravenous fluids, vasoactive medications, and possible mechanical circulatory support should be considered. Bedside echocardiography should be used at regular intervals to evaluate for pericardial effusion presence and growth. If the patient begins to have signs of tamponade physiology, emergent pericardiocentesis should be performed. Central venous access, usually femoral, should be obtained to allow for the autotransfusion of potentially large volumes of pericardial blood. If pericardiocentesis is unsuccessful, an emergent pericardial window may be warranted to prevent further hemodynamic collapse.

Polytetrafluoroethylene (PTFE)-covered stents are available on a humanitarian use basis and have reduced the need for emergency surgery and mortality in main branch vessel perforations.[19,20] In the past, covered stents had challenges with deliverability and required 7 French (F) or 8 F guide catheters. However, new generations of the PTFE stents such as the Papyrus stent (Biotronik) can often be delivered with the same 6 F guide catheter used for PCI. However, PTFE-covered stents remain bulkier than drug-eluting stents and less deliverable, so a second, larger guide catheter may be needed. In such cases, continued balloon hemostasis is maintained while the second guide catheter is advanced. Guide catheter engagement is alternated using a "ping-pong technique," whereby the 1st guide catheter with the occlusive balloon is disengaged to allow for the second guide to engage and send a coronary wire down into the perforated vessel as the occlusive balloon is momentarily deflated.[21] The PTFE-covered stent is then quickly advanced through the second guide catheter to the site of perforation and deployed following removal of the angioplasty balloon.[21] If an upsized single arterial access site is used, an 8F guide catheter will accommodate both a balloon and 2.5 to 3.0 mm PTFE-covered stent. After the patient has been stabilized and the perforation seems to be sealed angiographically, intracoronary imaging is recommended as the expansion of the PTFE-covered stent may require significant high-pressure postdilation, as restenosis and closure of PTFE stents occurs at a higher rate. Of note, side branch vessels near the perforation may be occluded with the PTFE-covered stent. Additionally, if proximal perforation occurs at a large branch site, emergent CABG may be preferable to covered stent deployment to avoid vessel closure.

Abrupt Vessel Closure

Abrupt vessel closure (AVC) is the most common coronary complication after PCI. Identifying the etiology of AVC is imperative as management differs substantially. The most common

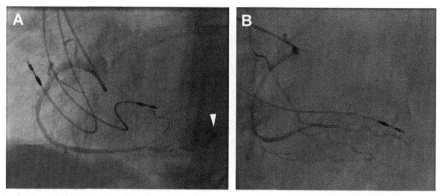

Fig. 1. Distal wire perforation is evident on contrast injection as a puff (*arrowhead*) (*A*). Following prolonged balloon inflation and reversal of anticoagulation, the perforation is no longer evident (*B*).

etiologies of AVC include dissection, no-reflow, intracoronary thrombus formation, air injection, and vasospasm. When AVC occurs the most imperative next step is to ensure wire position is not lost and that the coronary wire is intraluminal. If there is doubt regarding the intraluminal position of the wire, either a microcatheter can be advanced distally into the vessel for contrast injection or intravascular imaging can be used to confirm positioning.

In the case of dissection causing AVC (Fig. 3), if initial contrast injection shows the guidewire to be in a false lumen, careful advancement of a secondary guidewire is necessary. Importantly, it is possible that there is a partial subintimal guidewire passage, which, if not caught on intravascular imaging, could be suggested if a balloon cannot be advanced. Subintimal revascularization by balloon or stenting in this case carries a high risk of dissection propagation and perforation. Once intraluminal positioning is ensured, stenting to tack closed the false

lumen is typically successful in restoring luminal patency.

Slow- and no-reflow

Another important complication is that of the no-reflow or slow-flow phenomenon (Fig. 4), which consists of a persistent decrease in myocardial blood flow after the opening of a previously occluded or stenotic epicardial coronary artery.[22] The pathophysiology of no-reflow leading to AVC is multi-factorial due to a combination of endothelial damage, microembolization, and vasospasm leading to neutrophil plugging and microvascular dysfunction.[23] Direct ischemic injury to the distal tissue may also play a role as ischemic myocytes are edematous and can protrude into the intima and decrease flow. No-reflow occurs most commonly in those undergoing primary PCI for STEMI, atherectomy, or vein graft intervention. In the case of the saphenous vein graft, prevention is key with the use of a distal embolic protection device, which has been shown to have significant improvements in post-PCI flow.[24] Aspiration thrombectomy has no role in the treatment of no-reflow as the site of occlusion is in the microvasculature.[25,26] When the no-reflow phenomenon occurs, the primary mechanism of treatment is with intracoronary pharmacologic agents preferably selectively at the site of the no-reflow using a microcatheter. Although the use of intracoronary adenosine has some of the strongest evidence,[27] other agents including nitroprusside, nicardipine, and epinephrine have also been shown to be useful.[28,29]

Thrombus

If not completely occlusive sometimes thrombus can be identified as the cause of AVC. Again, after ensuring wire is intraluminal, multiple brief balloon inflations may be able to restore

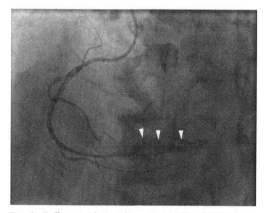

Fig. 2. Balloon and wire dissection during a chronic total occlusion intervention resulted in significant proximal dissection (*arrowheads*).

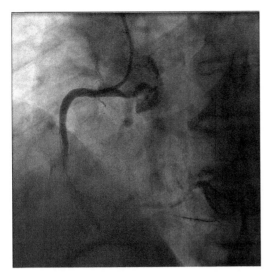

Fig. 3. After postdilatation of a large stent in a thrombotic right coronary artery (RCA) lesion, slow reflow is evident based on residual contrast in the distal RCA and branches.

effect may be prudent. Selective use of aspiration thrombectomy for large or persistent thrombus can be considered.[25,26] Thrombus should not be presumed to be the cause of occlusive vessel closure absent imaging evidence, as the administration of intravenous antiplatelet agents will increase the bleeding risk from emergency CABG.

Vasospasm
Extreme vasospasm may also lead to AVC. This can be difficult to differentiate between the other causes of AVC, but fortunately responds to vasodilators in a similar fashion to no-reflow. In such cases, intracoronary nitroglycerin can be given to aid antegrade flow. In some situations, especially in more distal, torturous smaller vessels, the coronary wire may also be contributing to the creating of pseudolesions as well as endothelial dysfunction leading to vasospasm. If confident that vasospasm is the cause of the reduced antegrade flow then pulling back the coronary wire may improve flow.

antegrade flow. Ensuring adequate anticoagulation is key after identifying intracoronary thrombus, first by noting the intravenous access is functioning properly as well as activating clotting times (ACT) are therapeutic. If the ACT is therapeutic, there is the possibility of agent resistance (usually heparin as this is the most commonly used anticoagulant), in which case switching to another agent such as bivalirudin maybe prudent. Administration of intravenous antiplatelet agents such as cangrelor or glycoprotein IIb/IIIa inhibitors is an additional option. Waiting a short period of time (20 minutes for example) for intravenous medication to take

Air embolism
Embolization of air can occur secondary to imperfect manifold or catheter preparation, resulting in air lock, in which a column of air is injected within the coronary artery preventing coronary flow into the coronary capillary network (Fig. 5). The key is prevention, as meticulous preparation of the manifold, tightening of valves and aggressive flushing of catheters make this extremely unlikely to occur. If the air embolus is more proximal, either guide catheter aspiration, microcatheter aspiration, or aspiration thrombectomy may be useful. 100% supplemental oxygen can facilitate the resolution of

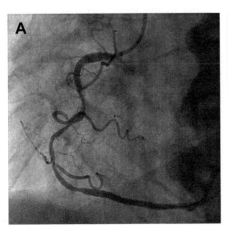
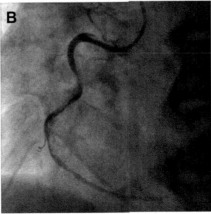

Fig. 4. A calcified and tortuous RCA (A) required a guide extension catheter to deliver a stent. The guide extension induced a dissection (B) that required stenting of the proximal to mid-RCA. Despite the initial recovery of distal perfusion, hyperacute stent thrombosis and acute vessel closure occurred.

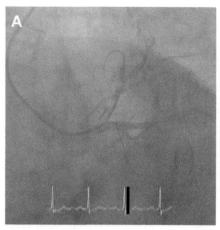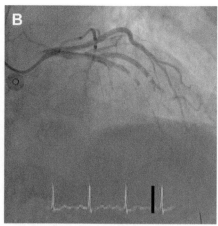

Fig. 5. Air emboli are evident during contrast injection during biplane angiography, proximally in the left anterior descending (LAD) artery in the LAO caudal (A) and then more distally in the mid-LAD and large diagonal in the AP cranial view (B).

air embolism via absorption. Additionally, a coronary wire or balloon can be advanced into the vessel to help reduce the surface tension of the air embolus, break the air embolus, and facilitate better absorption.

In all cases of AVC hemodynamic and electrical instability are real possibilities. Hypotension should be aggressively treated with fluid and vasopressors, while atropine should be used for bradycardia. This becomes particularly important when multiple rounds of intracoronary vasodilators are given for no-reflow. Given the risk of decompensation, preparations should be made for emergency CABG at the first detection of AVC, even if the complication initially seems manageable.

Device Embolization

Device embolization is a rare complication of PCI that occurs most commonly with the loss of a stent or guide-wire fragment within the coronary vasculature. Stent dislodgement occurs in approximately 0.32% of PCI based on a single-center study of more than 11,000 PCIs.[30]

Stent embolization occurs when an undeployed or incompletely deployed stent unintentionally comes off the intracoronary balloon. There are a handful of situations in which this occurs: (1) a stent is withdrawn into a noncoaxial guide catheter (after failing to be advanced to the intended location for example) leading to the stent to be stripped off the balloon by the edge of the guide, (2) passing a stent across another recently placed stent leading to the stent being stripped off the balloon, and (3) attempted passage of a stent through a tortuous

or calcified lesion causing the stent to become stuck (Fig. 6).

Prevention is again key for preventing stent embolization. Optimal guide catheter selection to ensure coaxial alignment reduces case complications and improves deliverability. Additionally, adequate lesion preparation, whether with serial predilatation or plaque modification, can prevent stent stripping. Identifying stent deformation before embolization is key. When there are unexpected difficulties in stent advancement, the stent should be gently retracted into the guide catheter and removed to evaluate the possibility of stent deformation.

There exist multiple strategies for recovering a loss sent.[31] If the stent remains on the coronary guide wire, a small angioplasty balloon (1.25 mm or 1.5 mm) can sometimes be passed into or distal to the stent and then inflated, resulting in the capture of the stent and retrieval into the guide catheter. If the stent cannot be retrieved into the guide catheter, because the guide is not coaxial for example, one can consider bringing the stent to the tip of the guide catheter and removing the entire ensemble as a unit. This, however, puts the ostium of the vessel at risk of damage. Another technique involves advancing a secondary coronary wire alongside the embolized stent through a stent strut, twist the wires together, and retract the stent. Gooseneck-type or other intracoronary snares can be considered to attempt to retrieve a loss stent. If attempts for retrieval are unsuccessful, an attempt at trying to pass a small balloon into the stent and inflating, followed by larger serial balloons to fully deploy the stent in

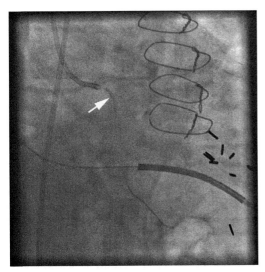

Fig. 6. A stent (*arrow*) became dislodged from its balloon within a calcified and tortuous LCx artery, possibly against the guide edge. Manual traction with a snare anchoring the stent was successful in retrieving the stent.

the location of loss is an option. Unfortunately, due to stent deformation passing a balloon into the stent may not be possible. At this point, it may be necessary to consider balloon crushing the stent against the arterial wall or deploying an additional stent alongside the embolized one. During all of these strategies, it is pivotal to ensure that the patient has adequate anticoagulation to reduce the likelihood of thrombus formation. Ultimately, AVC may occur, and at this point, emergent CABG should be considered.

When the embolized item is a piece of guidewire, retrieval may be more difficult compared with a stent based on the size of the retained object. Nonetheless, addressing the retained piece of guidewire is important as distal embolization could lead to perforation and possible tamponade.[32] Retrieval can be achieved by sending another coronary wire down and attempting to wrap the wires to remove together as a unit or using a snare. Depending on the position of the retained fragment, stenting to seal the fragment against the coronary wall to prevent late distal migration can be considered.

Rotational Atherectomy Burr Entrapment
The usage of rotational atherectomy has grown to address calcified coronary artery lesions. However, careful consideration should be given to when to use rotational atherectomy to prepare a lesion given serious complications including coronary dissection or perforation, no-reflow phenomenon, vasospasm, or distal

embolization.[33] Burr entrapment is a unique complication occurring in 0.5% to 1% of cases.[33–36] Entrapment occurs when a burr is embedded in severe stenosis, preventing both advancement and retrieval, usually in tortuous vessels. Prevention is usually achieved by advancing using gentle pecking motions, short runs ensuring the burr does not dive distally, avoidance of decelerations greater than 5000 rpms, and ensuring a maximum burr-to-artery ratio of 0.5 to 0.6.[32]

If entrapment occurs, manual system pullback should be attempted with Dynaglide rotation on. However, only gentle traction should be used to avoid vessel damage or burr shaft fracture. If this does not work, then a separate guide catheter should be engaged (via secondary arterial access) to allow for a separate guidewire advancement and serial balloon dilations next to the burr to facilitate the release of the entrapped burr. Other techniques include dissembling the Rotablator apparatus to expose the burr shaft allowing a percutaneous snare to be advanced proximal to the burr and providing gentle traction with removal.[37] Countertraction with a guide extension "child-in-a-mother catheter" can also be attempted to allow for gentle traction without the need for surgical intervention.[38]

SUMMARY

PCI remains a safe and effective treatment of coronary artery disease. As advancing technology allows for interventions on increasingly more complex lesions in older patients, the potential for complications increases. Prevention of coronary complications via meticulous attention to detail and technique is vital, but education, rescue equipment, and cath laboratory team drills on potential complications are necessary for these rare events. When the inevitable complication occurs, rapid identification and management can be lifesaving.

CLINICAL CASE PEARLS

- Once grade III coronary perforation is identified, immediate proximal balloon inflation is critical while the cath laboratory team rapidly mobilizes medications (fluid, vasoactive support) and equipment (additional access site preparation, covered stent, and so forth) while continuously evaluating the patient's hemodynamics.

- Management of coronary perforations is based on location, with distal vessel and septal perforator coronary perforations often responding to a combination of proximal balloon inflation, anticoagulation reversal, and embolization (subcutaneous fat, coils, beads, or thrombin).
- Once no-reflow is identified as the cause of abrupt vessel closure, multiple rounds of directed intracoronary vasodilators have the best evidence for the restoration of intracoronary flow as long as blood pressure permits.
- Use of manual aspiration thrombectomy is typically ineffective in no-reflow, but can be considered in vessel closure due to large thrombus burden.
- While an embolized stent can be retrieved via the use of distal inflation of a small angioplasty balloon, wrapping a coronary wire through stent struts, or an intracoronary snare, depending on the location of the embolized stent, deployment of the stent should be considered.

DISCLOSURE

Dr D.M. Tehrani has no disclosures. Dr A.H. Seto has research grants from Philips and Acist, honoraria from Janssen, Acist, Terumo, and consulting fees from Medicare and Medtronic.

REFERENCES

1. Johnson LW, Lozner EC, Johnson S, et al. Coronary arteriography 1984-1987: a report of the registry of the society for cardiac angiography and interventions.I. results and complications. Cathet Cardiovasc Diagn 1989;17(1):5–10.
2. Latif F, Kleiman NS, Cohen DJ, et al. In-Hospital and 1-Year Outcomes Among Percutaneous Coronary Intervention Patients With Chronic Kidney Disease in the Era of Drug-Eluting Stents: A Report From the EVENT (Evaluation of Drug Eluting Stents and Ischemic Events) Registry. JACC Cardiovasc Interv 2009;2:37–45.
3. Cook S, Wenaweser P, Togni M, et al. Incomplete stent apposition and very late stent thrombosis after drug-eluting stent implantation. Circulation 2007;115:2426–34.
4. Alkhouli M, Alqahtani F, Tarabishy A, et al. Incidence, Predictors, and Outcomes of Acute Ischemic Stroke Following Percutaneous Coronary Intervention. JACC Cardiovasc Interv 2019;12(15): 1497–506.
5. Kutcher MA, Klein LW, Fang-Shu O, et al. Percutaneous Coronary Interventions in Facilities Without Cardiac Surgery on Site: A Report from the National Cardiovascular Data Registry. J Am Coll Cardiol 2019;30:16–24.
6. Anderson HV, Shaw RE, Brindis RG, et al. A contemporary overview of percutaneous coronary interventions. The American college of cardiology national cardiovascular data registry (ACC-NCDR). J Am Coll Cardiol 2002;39(7):1096–103.
7. Peterson ED, Dai D, Delong ER, et al. Contemporary Mortality Risk Prediction for Percutaneous Coronary Intervention: Results from 588,398 Procedures in the National Cardiovascular Data Registry. J Am Coll Cardiol 2010; 55(18):1923–32.
8. Castro-Dominguez SY, Wang U, Minges KE, et al. Predicting In-Hospital Mortality in Patients Undergoing Percutaneous Coronary Intervention. J Am Coll Cardiol 2021;78(3):216–29.
9. Shimony A, Joseph L, Mottillo S, et al. Coronary artery perforation during percutaneous coronary intervention: a systematic review and meta-analysis. Can J Cardiol 2011;27:843–50.
10. Kinnaird T, Kwok CS, Kontopantelis E, et al. Incidence, determinants and outcomes of coronary perforation during percutaneous coronary intervention in the United Kingdom between 2006 and 2013. An analysis of 527121 cases from the British Cardiovascular Intervention Society Database. Circ Cardiovasc Interv 2016;9:e003449.
11. Dippel EJ, Kereiakes DJ, Tramuta DA, et al. Coronary perforation during percutaneous coronary intervention in the era of abciximab platelet glycoprotein IIb/IIIa blockade: an algorithm for percutaneous management. Catheter Cardiovasc Interv 2001;52:279–86.
12. Kiernan TJ, Yan BP, Ruggeiro N, et al. Coronary artery perforations in the contemporary interventional era. J Interv Cardiol 2009;22:350–3.
13. Brilakis ES. Manual of Coronary Chronic Total Occlusion Interventions: A Step-by-Step Approach 1st Edition, 2014.
14. De Marco F, Balcells J, Lefèvre T, et al. Delayed and recurrent cardiac tamponade following distal coronary perforation of hydrophilic guidewires during coronary intervention. J Invasive Cardiol 2008;20:E150–3.
15. Aleong G, Jimenez-Quevedo P, Alfonso F. Collagen embolization for the successful treatment of a distal coronary artery perforation. Catheter Cardiovasc Interv 2009;73:332–5.
16. Gaxiola E, Browne KF. Coronary artery perforation repair using microcoil embolization. Cathet Cardiovasc Diagn 1998;43:474–6.
17. Shirakabe A, Takano H, Nakamura S, et al. Coronary perforation during percutaneous coronary intervention. Int Heart J 2007;48:1–9.

18. Lansky AJ, Yang Y-M, Khan Y, et al. Treatment of coronary artery perforations complicating percutaneous coronary intervention with a polytetrafluoroethylene-covered stent graft. Am J Cardiol 2006;98:370–4.

19. Gruberg I, Pinnow E, Flood R, et al. Incidence, management, and outcome of coronary artery perforation during percutaneous coronary intervention. Am J Cardiol 2000;86:680–2.

20. Gunning MG, Williams IL, Jewitt DE, et al. Coronary artery perforation during percutaneous intervention: incidence and outcome. Heart 2002;88:495–8.

21. Ben-Gal Y, Weisz G, Collins MB, et al. Dual catheter technique for the treatment of severe coronary artery perforations. Catheter Cardiovasc Interv 2009; 75:708–12.

22. Rezkalla SH, Kloner RA. No-reflow phenomenon. Circulation 2002;105:656–62.

23. Abbo KM, Dooris M, Glazier S, et al. Features and outcome of no-reflow after percutaneous coronary intervention. Am J Cardiol 1995;75:778–82.

24. Sturm E, Goldberg D, Goldberg S. Embolic protection devices in saphenous vein graft and native vessel percutaneous intervention: a review. Curr Cardiol Rev 2012;8(3):192–9.

25. Frobert O, Lagerqvist B, Olivercrona GK, et al. Thrombus Aspiration during ST-Segment Elevation Myocardial Infarction. N Engl J Med 2013;369:1587–97.

26. Jolly SS, Cairns JA, Yusuf S, et al. Randomized Trial of Primary PCI with or without Routine Manual Thrombectomy. N Engl J Med 2015;372:1389–98.

27. Micari A, Belcik TA, Balcells EA, et al. Improvement in microvascular reflow and reduction of infarct size with adenosine in patients undergoing primary coronary stenting. Am J Cardiol 2005;96:1410–5.

28. Rezkalla SH, Dharmashankar KC, Abdalrahman IB. No-reflow phenomenon following percutaneous coronary intervention for acute myocardial infarction: incidence, outcome and effect of pharmacologic therapy. J Interv Cardiol 2010;23:429–43.

29. Aksu T, Guler TE, Colak A, et al. Intracoronary epinephrine in the treatment of refractory noreflow after primary percutaneous coronary intervention: a retrospective study. BMC Cardiovasc Disord 2015; 15:10.

30. Brilakis ES, Best PJM, Elesber AA, et al. Incidence, retrieval methods, and outcomes of stent loss during percutaneous coronary intervention. Catheter Cardiovasc Interv 2005;65:333–40.

31. Bolte J, Neumann U, Pfafferott C, et al. Incidence, management, and outcome of stent loss during intracoronary stenting. Am J Cardiol 2001;88:565–7.

32. Hartzler GO, Rutherford BD, McConahay DR. Retained percutaneous transluminal coronary angioplasty equipment components and their management. Am J Cardiol 1987;60:1260–4.

33. Tomey MI, Kini AS, Sharma SK. Current status of rotational atherectomy. JACC Cardiovasc Interv 2014;7(4):345–53.

34. Abdel-Wahab M, Richardt G, Joachim Buttner H, et al. High-speed rotational atherectomy before paclitaxel-eluting stent implantation in complex calcified coronary lesions: the randomized ROTAXUS (Rotational Atherectomy Prior to Taxus Stent Treatment for Complex Native Coronary Artery Disease) trial. J Am Coll Cardiol Intv 2013;6: 10–9.

35. Sulimov DS, Abdel-Wahab M, Toelg R, et al. Stuck rotablator: the nightmare of rotational atherectomy. EuroIntervention 2013;9:251–8.

36. Kaneda H, Saito S, Hosokawa G, et al. Trapped rotablator: Kokesi phenomenon. Catheter Cardiovasc Interv 2000;49:82–4.

37. Prasan AM, Patel M, Pitney MR, et al. Disassembly of a rotablator: Getting out of a trap. Catheter Cardiovasc Interv 2003;59:463–5.

38. Cunnington M, Egred M. GuideLiner, a child in- a-mother catheter for successful retrieval of an entrapped rotablator burr. Catheter Cardiovasc Interv 2012;79:271–3.

Patient Selection for Protected Percutaneous Coronary Intervention
Who Benefits the Most?

Seung-Hyun Kim, MD*, Stefan Baumann, MD,
Michael Behnes, MD, Martin Borggrefe, MD,
Ibrahim Akin, MD

KEYWORDS

• High-risk-PCI • Protected PCI • MCS devices • IABP • pLVAD • LAAD • VA-ECMO

KEY POINTS

- Definition of protected percutaneous coronary intervention (PCI) and hemodynamic impact of diverse mechanical circulatory support devices.
- Clinical criteria for patient selection for protected PCI.
- Procedure-related criteria for patient selection for protected PCI.
- Algorithm and scoring system for patient selection for protected PCI.

INTRODUCTION

A development of percutaneous coronary intervention (PCI) with device innovation, novel skills, and effective antiproliferative medications allows for addressing increasingly complex coronary artery disease (CAD).[1] However, simultaneously, patients are presenting nowadays with higher rates of comorbidities and more complex CAD, which may lead to a lower physiologic tolerance for complex PCI. This patient group would be poor candidates for coronary artery bypass grafting (CABG) because of the high risk of surgical morbidity and mortality.[2]

As an alternative approach, the concept of so-called "protected PCI" has been developed, in which mechanical circulatory support (MCS) is used for the PCI in this high-risk patient group. The purpose of MCS is to provide hemodynamic support for complex PCI, and concurrently to reduce left ventricular systolic work and

myocardial oxygen demand while maintaining systemic and coronary perfusion.[3] Currently, the following devices are available for MCS: intra-aortic balloon pump (IABP), percutaneous left ventricular assist devices (pLVAD), left atrial to aorta assist devices (LAAD), and veno-arterial extracorporeal membrane oxygenation (VA-ECMO). Using MCS devices in combination with an optimal selection of patients and devices would potentially improve the success rate of interventional procedures and clinical outcomes in these high-risk patients.[4,5]

However, since multiple treatment modalities are available and the precise definition of "high-risk patients" has not yet been established, it is still not clearly determined who benefits the most from protected PCI and which MCS device offers the best result in each clinical scenario. Hence, this review aims to provide practical approaches for the appropriate selection of patients and MCS device types by outlining

This article originally appeared in Cardiology Clinics, Volume 38, Issue 4, November 2020.
First Department of Medicine, University Medical Centre Mannheim (UMM), Faculty of Medicine Mannheim, University of Heidelberg, European Center for AngioScience (ECAS), and DZHK (German Center for Cardiovascular Research) Partner Site Heidelberg/Mannheim, Theodor-Kutzer-Ufer 1-3, Mannheim 68167, Germany
* Corresponding author.
E-mail address: seung-hyun.kim@umm.de

current clinical data that assess utility of diverse MCS devices in high-risk patients undergoing protected PCI.

DEFINITION OF PROTECTED PERCUTANEOUS CORONARY INTERVENTION

The evolution of PCI techniques has enhanced the number of patients eligible for PCI of complex coronary lesions, for example, unprotected left main coronary stenosis, heavily calcified stenosis, and chronic total occlusion.[6] Nevertheless, each aspect of PCI, beginning from guide catheter engagement and ending with balloon inflation and stent deployment, is associated with potential risk of vascular damage and impairment of myocardial perfusion. Especially, patients with more complex CAD evaluated by higher SYNTAX (Synergy between Percutaneous Coronary Intervention with Taxus and Cardiac Surgery) score and concurrent higher surgical mortality assessed by higher STS (the Society of Thoracic Surgeons) score would not be suitable for either PCI[7] or for CABG.[8] Specifically, the PCI in patients with reduced coronary perfusion gradients between coronary arterioles and venules could cause a severe myocardial ischemia and consequently ischemia-triggered cardiac arrhythmias or further depression of an already impaired left ventricular ejection fraction (LVEF), leading to circulatory collapse and cardiac arrest.[9,10] Furthermore, complete or sufficient revascularization could not be guaranteed due to hemodynamic instability during the procedures. To avoid this fatal consequence, so-called protected PCI using MCS device as an alternative strategy for safely achieving complete revascularization has been used for more than 25 years.[11] The purpose of MCS is to decrease myocardial oxygen demand by reducing left ventricular volume (preload) and pressure (afterload) during high-risk PCI.[12] Another goal of MCS is to achieve sufficient cardiac output to maintain myocardial, cerebral, renal, mesenteric, and peripheral tissue perfusion, thereby preventing systemic shock syndrome. In addition, the use of appropriate MCS devices can provide sufficient time to safely perform high-risk PCI with optimal results in this patient group who would not otherwise tolerate complete revascularization.[13]

HEMODYNAMIC IMPACT OF MECHANICAL CIRCULATORY SUPPORT DEVICES

Currently, diverse types of percutaneous MCS with different characteristics and hemodynamic impact are available for high-risk PCI.[14] First, IABP supports hemodynamic circulation by inflating and deflating the balloon based on an electrocardiogram (ECG) or pressure triggers.[15] The balloon inflating occurs with the onset of diastole timed to the middle of the T-wave on ECG. Thereafter, the balloon deflates rapidly at the beginning of left ventricular systole corresponding to the pear of the R-wave on ECG. The IABP decreases myocardial oxygen demand by reducing left ventricular afterload, and increases coronary artery perfusion by enhancing diastolic blood pressure. However, there are some functional limitations of IABP. Whereas mean arterial pressure and coronary blood flow are increased by using IABP, it offers only modest left ventricular unloading defined by reducing left ventricular volume and pressure (Fig. 1A). A stable electrical rhythm is also a prerequisite for the optimal hemodynamic effect from IABP, because IABP works depending on the surface ECG. The further limitations of IABP are dependence on native left ventricular function, balloon capacity, and accurate timing of balloon inflation and deflation.[16]

Second, the pLVAD is a continuous nonpulsatile microaxial screw pump deployed into the left ventricle across the aortic valve to pump blood from the left ventricle to the ascending aorta.[17] In this way, the pLVAD increases forward flow to the ascending aorta and mean arterial pressure. At the same time, it reduces myocardial oxygen demand and pulmonary capillary wedge pressure.[18] In contrast to IABP, the hemodynamic support from pLVAD is dependent neither on the native left ventricular function of patients nor on electrical stability due to its direct continuous propelling of blood from the left ventricle to the ascending aorta. The pLVAD leads to a remarkable unloading of the left ventricle by reducing left ventricular systolic and diastolic pressures, left ventricular volumes, and stroke volume (Fig. 1B). In case of biventricular failure or unstable ventricular arrhythmias, concomitantly using a right ventricular assist device should be considered to maintain left ventricular preload and optimal hemodynamic support from pLVAD.

The LAAD is one of the MCS devices that extracorporeally pumps blood from the left atrium via a transseptally placed left atrial cannula to the iliofemoral arterial system, thereby bypassing the left ventricle.[17] The bypass of blood from the left atrium induces indirectly optimal left ventricular unload at a similar level to pLVAD that enables direct unloading of the left ventricle (see Fig. 1B). By this means, the LAAD reduces wall stress and myocardial

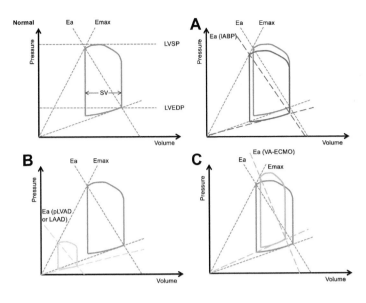

Fig. 1. Hemodynamic imbalance in acute myocardial infarction and cardiogenic shock, and hemodynamic impact of various MCS devices are illustrated by the pressure-volume loop. The normal pressure-volume loop is shown in blue. Emax representing a load-independent left ventricular contractility is defined as the maximal slope of the end-systolic pressure-volume point under various loading conditions, known as the end-systolic pressure-volume relationship. Effective arterial elastance (Ea) is a component of left ventricular afterload and is defined as the ratio of left ventricular systolic pressure (LVSP) and stroke volume (SV). (A) Pressure-volume loop in using IABP demonstrates a mildly decreased left ventricular end-diastolic pressure (LVEDP) and LVSP, leading to decreased an Ea. (B) Pressure-volume loop with pLVAD and LAAD shows a substantially decreased LVEDP, LVSP, and SV. The net effect is a pronounced reduction of left ventricular preload and afterload. (C) Pressure-volume loop with VA-ECMO without left ventricular venting indicates a decreased SV, whereas LVEDP und LVSP are significantly increased with a net effect of substantial increase of left ventricular afterload. (Adapted from Rihal CS, Naidu SS, Givertz MM, et al. 2015 SCAI/ACC/HFSA/STS Clinical Expert Consensus Statement on the Use of Percutaneous Mechanical Circulatory Support Devices in Cardiovascular Care: Endorsed by the American Heart Assocation, the Cardiological Society of India, and Sociedad Latino Americana de Cardiologia Intervencion; Affirmation of Value by the Canadian Association of Interventional Cardiology-Association Canadienne de Cardiologie d'intervention. J Am Coll Cardiol. 2015;65(19): e7-e26.)

oxygen demand.[19] However, the need for a transseptal puncture is an important obstacle for clinical use of LAAD.

Finally, VA-ECMO provides both oxygenation and circulation. A venous cannula drains deoxygenated blood into a membrane oxygenator for gas exchange, and oxygenated blood is subsequently infused into the patient via an arterial cannula. VA-ECMO provides systemic circulatory support with flows sometimes exceeding 6 L/min depending on cannula sizes. However, it can significantly increase afterload on the left ventricle (Fig. 1C), thereby potentially reducing left ventricular stroke volume, increasing myocardial oxygen demand, and necessitating "venting" of the left ventricle by concomitant IABP or pLVAD.[20,21] In contrast to conventional VA-ECMO, the novel pulsatile ECMO triggered by ECG provides a more sufficient coronary perfusion with less increase in afterload.

CLINICAL CRITERIA FOR PATIENT SELECTION FOR PROTECTED PERCUTANEOUS CORONARY INTERVENTION

Recently, the clinical practice guidelines recommend consideration of the use of these devices in the setting of high-risk PCI.[3] To avoid underutilization or overutilization of MCS devices during high-risk PCI and to minimize the associated risk, however, a proper patient selection is paramount. Based on patient inclusion criteria adopted in prior various studies assessing utility of protected PCI, the following factors are generally considered as major criteria in patient selection for protected PCI[22] (Table 1). First, one of these factors is the lesion characteristic that determines the complexity of PCI reflecting the technical perspectives and the potential risk of complications. It includes unprotected left main coronary stenosis, distal left main bifurcation stenosis, multivessel disease with high SYNTAX score (≥33), myocardial jeopardy score (≥8/12), last remaining coronary conduit, heavily calcified lesions (type C lesion), and chronic total occlusions. Shamekhi and colleagues[23] revealed that patients undergoing protected PCI with pLVAD achieved more often a complete revascularization without the occurrence of cardiac death at 30 days of follow-up compared with patients undergoing unprotected PCI despite a higher SYNTAX score (45% vs 36%, P = .07) and more often complex left main bifurcation lesions (71% vs 29%). Moreover, a similar major adverse cardiac event rate (MACE) at 1 year of

Table 1
Clinical criteria for patient selection for protected PCI

Lesion characteristic	Unprotected left main coronary stenosis
	Distal left main bifurcation stenosis
	Multivessel disease with higher SYNTAX score ($\geq$33) or myocardial jeopardy ($\geq$8/12)
	Last remaining coronary conduit
	Heavily calcified lesions (type C lesion)
	Chronic total occlusions
Severe decompensated heart failure	LVEF ($\leq$30–40%)
	NYHA classification III-IV
	Killip classification II-IV
	Electrical instability (eg, ventricular tachycardia)
Patient comorbidities with higher STS-score or EuroSCORE	Increased age (>75 y)
	Chronic obstructive lung disease
	Chronic kidney disease
	Peripheral vascular disease
	Diabetes mellitus
Hemodynamic parameters	Cardiac index (<2.2 L/min per m^2)
	Pulmonary capillary wedge pressure (>15 mm Hg)
	Mean pulmonary artery pressure (>30 mm Hg)

Abbreviations: LVEF, left ventricular ejection fraction; NYHA, New York Heart Association; PCI, percutaneous coronary intervention; STS, Society of Thoracic Surgeons; SYNTAX, synergy between percutaneous coronary intervention with taxus and cardiac surgery.

follow-up between both groups was shown despite severe basic characteristics of the protected PCI group. These are consistent with results of another study, in which patients undergoing protected PCI with pLVAD had also a decreased rate of residual stenosis and increased rate of procedural success compared with patients with unprotected PCI. The short-term and long-term outcomes in terms of MACE were also similar despite the significantly higher SYNTAX score in the protected PCI group (33% vs 24%, P<.01).[24] The extended randomized BCIS-1 trial (Balloon Pump-Assisted Coronary Intervention Study) demonstrated that protected PCI using IABP reduced relatively a long-term all-cause mortality in patients with higher myocardial jeopardy score ($\geq$8) compared with the unprotected PCI group.[25]

Second, protected PCI might be proper for patients with severe decompensated heart failure with reduced LVEF ($\leq$30–40%), New York Heart Association (NYHA) classification III-IV, Killip classification II–IV, or electrical instability (eg, ventricular tachycardia). Ameloot and colleagues[5] showed that patients with severely reduced LVEF (median 24%) and concomitant

higher SYNTAX score (median 33) have benefited from protected PCI using pLVAD in terms of survival rate. In a registry trial involving patients with decreased LVEF (mean 31%) and higher SYNTAX score (median 37), it was shown that protected PCI with pLVAD significantly improved LVEF and NYHA class of these high-risk patients.[26] In the PROTECT II trial (Prospective Randomized Clinical Trial of Hemodynamic Support with Impella 2.5 vs Intra-Aortic Balloon Pump in Patients undergoing High-Risk Percutaneous Coronary Intervention) involving patients with reduced LVEF (<30%–35%) and concurrent unprotected left main stenosis or 3-vessel disease, patients undergoing protected PCI with pLVAD have achieved a more hemodynamic stabilization.[27] Thereby, the frequent occurrence of complete revascularization and the associated reduction of MACE in the protected PCI group might be explained.

Third, patient comorbidities, including increased age (>75 years), chronic obstructive lung disease, chronic kidney disease, peripheral arterial disease, and diabetes mellitus, should be evaluated by STS-score or EuroSCORE when selecting patients for protected PCI.

Patients with higher comorbidities assessed by higher STS-score or EuroSCORE could not be suitable for surgical revascularization due to the underlying increased expected risk of mortality and morbidity,.[28–30] In a multicenter registry study, it was shown that protected PCI using pLVAD might be a safe and effective alternative approach to revascularize coronary lesions in patients with higher SYNTAX score (median 32) and concurrent higher logistic EuroSCORE (median 14.7).[31] Another study demonstrated also the safety of both pLVAD and LAAD for protected PCI, especially in patients with complex coronary anatomy and reduced LVEF (median 31%) who were rejected for CABG because of higher mortality risk (median STS-score of 4.2%).[32] Recently, Baumann and colleagues[33] demonstrated in a multicenter registry study that patients undergoing protected PCI with pLVAD due to both higher SYNTAX score (median 33) and higher EuroSCORE II (median 7.2%) had acceptable clinical results at 180 days of follow-up regarding MACE (22%) and all-cause mortality (18%).

Finally, hemodynamic parameters are also regarded as key factors, especially reduced cardiac index (<2.2 L/min per m^2), increased pulmonary capillary wedge pressure (>15 mm Hg), and mean pulmonary artery pressure (>30 mm Hg). The safety and efficacy of IABP and LAAD for protected PCI could be demonstrated in a randomized study including patients with a cardiac index less than 2.1 L/min per m^2 indicating an onset of cardiogenic shock.[34] In contrast, however, no study could clearly demonstrate the mortality advantage of MCS devices in patients with already manifested severe cardiogenic shock despite improvement in hemodynamic and metabolic parameters by using MCS devices.[35–38]

PROCEDURE-RELATED CRITERIA FOR PATIENT SELECTION FOR PROTECTED PERCUTANEOUS CORONARY INTERVENTION

In addition to the previously mentioned clinical criteria, procedure-related factors also should be considered in patient selection for protected PCI to reduce procedure-related complications and thus to improve clinical outcomes (Table 2). These depend basically on the selection of MCS devices due to the different implantation techniques and operating mechanisms.[39] The factor that is independent of types of MCS devices is a pathologic peripheral vessel condition, such as tortuosity and/or peripheral arterial disease.

This factor does not actually represent an absolute contraindication for the implantation of MCS devices of all types.[3] However, it is associated with increased risk of limb ischemia or mechanical malfunction of MCS devices.[40] Especially in patients with known peripheral arterial disease, severity of disease should be assessed by imaging diagnostics, such as duplex ultrasonography or even computed tomography angiography to determine the appropriate access vessel for insertion of the device's sheath. In this regard, for example, patients with severe peripheral arterial disease or tortuosity in iliofemoral vessels could benefit more from pLVAD with an axillary access than from the other devices.[22]

In addition, the indication of protected PCI should be carefully evaluated in patients with aortic valve disease (ie, aortic regurgitation or aortic stenosis).[41] Even with mild aortic regurgitation, all types of MCS devices could increase significantly the volume of regurgitation due to increased aortic pressure, leading to further dilatation of aorta and left ventricle and consequently severe decompensating hemodynamics.[42,43] Specifically, in case of pLVAD in patients with aortic regurgitation, an optimal forward flow mediated by pLVAD could be not guaranteed due to the lack of a competent valve separating between the left ventricle and aorta.[44] Moreover, patients with an aortic stenosis will be also poorly served by pLVAD because of difficult placement caused by the aortic stenosis and an increased risk of thromboembolism as well as rupture. Therefore, assessment of aortic valve using transthoracic (TTE) or transesophageal echocardiography (TEE) before protected PCI is recommended.

The presence of thrombus is also one of criteria that should be excluded by TTE or TEE before the planed protected PCI using particularly pLVAD or LAAD.[44] An ingestion of left ventricular clot in pLVAD commonly leads to shutdown of the device. The likelihood of clot ingestion resulting in embolization is extremely unlikely; however, a mobile thrombus represents a risk for systemic embolization with any left ventricular catheter placement. When using LAAD, thrombus in the left atrium could lead to the shutdown of the LAAD or/and a systemic embolization, such as an ischemic stroke, mesenteric ischemia, and renal infarction. Hence, preprocedural visualization of the left ventricle and atrium excluding the presence of thrombus is advisable.

In protected PCI with pLVAD, LAAD, or VA-ECMO, an adequate anticoagulation is indispensable to prevent thrombus formation that leads to malfunctions of devices and systemic

Table 2
Procedure-related criteria for selection of patients and MCS devices for protected PCI

	Criterium	Available MCS Devices
Peripheral vessel condition assessed by duplex ultrasonography or CTA	Iliofemoral tortuosity	Axillary pLVAD, IABP
	Iliofemoral peripheral arterial disease	
Aortic valve disease assessed by TTE or TEE	Aortic regurgitation	No devices recommended
	Aortic stenosis	IABP, LAAD, VA-ECMO
Presence of thrombus assessed by TTE or TEE	Thrombus in left ventricle	IABP, LAAD, VA-ECMO
	Thrombus in left atrium	IABP, VA-ECMO
Contraindication for anticoagulation	Thrombocytopenia	IABP
	Liver synthesis disorder	
	von Willebrand disease	
	Disseminated intravascular coagulation	

Abbreviations: CTA, computed tomography angiography; IABP, intra-aortic balloon pump; LAAD, left atrial to aorta assist devices; MCS, mechanical circulatory support; PCI, percutaneous coronary intervention; pLVAD, percutaneous left ventricular assist devices; TEE, transesophageal echocardiography; TTE, transthoracic echocardiography; VA-ECMO, veno-arterial extracorporeal membrane oxygenation.

thromboembolism.[45] In this context, patients with hemorrhagic diathesis, for example, thrombocytopenia, liver synthesis disorder, von Willebrand disease, or disseminated intravascular coagulation, might benefit rather from protected PCI using IABP instead of pLVAD, LAAD or VA-ECMO.

ALGORITHM AND SCORING SYSTEM FOR PATIENT SELECTION FOR PROTECTED PERCUTANEOUS CORONARY INTERVENTION

According to recommendations of European Society of Cardiology 2017, IABP insertion should be considered in patients with hemodynamic instability or cardiogenic shock due to mechanical complications (Class IIa), whereas no other devices are recommended.[46] In patients with acute myocardial infarction complicated by cardiogenic shock, short-term MCS may be considered regardless of device types (Class IIb). According to the guidelines of American College of Cardiology/American Heart Association/Society for Cardiovascular Angiography and Interventions, elective insertion of an appropriate MCS device as an adjunct to PCI has been recommended in carefully selected high-risk patients who have a vessel subtending a large territory on a background of severely depressed left ventricular function, unprotected left main, or last remaining conduit (Class IIa).[47]

So far, however, no established algorithm or scoring system reflecting all clinical and procedure-related criteria has been developed that can be generally used in patient selection for protected PCI to prevent underestimating or overestimating. Werner and colleagues[48] suggested in their expert consensus an algorithm for patient selection for protected PCI based on coronary complexity, LVEF, cardiac index, and comorbidities; however, herewith also no procedure-related criteria were considered when selecting patients for protected PCI. In the algorithm suggested by Atkinson and colleagues,[22] an evaluation of femoral vessel was reflected to determine the access vessel for inserting MCS devices, but no other procedure-related factors were described in detail. A single-center registry by McCabe[49] evaluating a proposed scoring system to guide patient selection for protected PCI is ongoing, and findings regarding the adequacy of these characteristics to predict efficacy and safety of upfront protected PCI are still pending (Fig. 2). Based on the previously proposed algorithms, Fig. 3 suggests a practical approach for patient selection for protected PCI depending on the clinical and technical aspects. To improve efficacy and safety of protected PCI in these high-risk patients exhibiting higher mortality, further clinical studies should be conducted to develop a universal reliable algorithm to select appropriate patients for protected PCI.

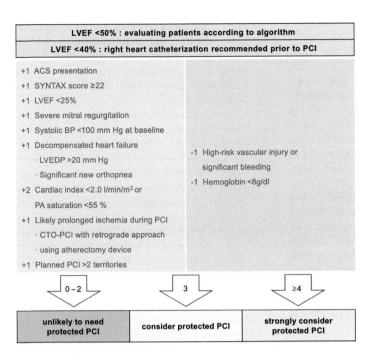

Fig. 2. Proposed scoring system based on clinical factors for optimal patient selection for protected PCI. ACS, acute coronary syndrome; BP, blood pressure; CI, cardiac index; CTO, chronic total occlusion; LVEDP, left ventricular end-diastolic pressure; PA, pulmonary artery. (Adapted from McCabe JM. Hemodynamic support for CTO PCI: who, when & how. Presented at Transcatheter Cardiovascular Therapeutics (TCT). September 21-25, 2018, San Diego, California.)

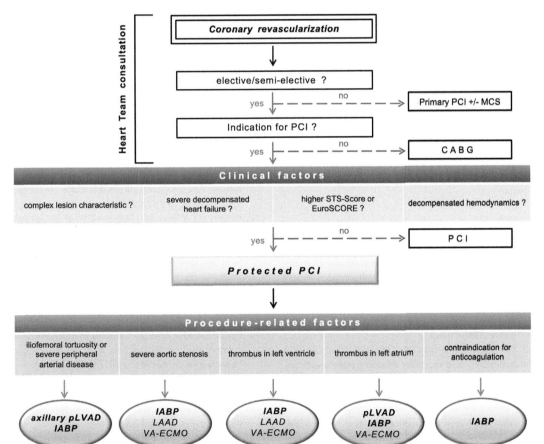

Fig. 3. Proposed practical approach for patient selection for protected PCI depending on the clinical and procedure-related factors. IABP or pLVAD should be preferred for protected PCI if there are no negative procedure-related factors for their use.

SUMMARY

Protected PCI represents one of the most advanced PCI types using several MCS devices to maintain sufficient cardiac output and reduce myocardial oxygen demand in high-risk patients who would not otherwise tolerate complete revascularization of complex coronary lesions. However, a precise selection of patients for protected PCI based on various clinical criteria is imperative to achieve hemodynamic and prognostic benefit in this patient group with higher morbidity and mortality burden. Moreover, the use of MCS devices for protected PCI should be also strictly individualized based on procedure-related factors to prevent device-associated complications. Further registry and randomized trials should be conducted to establish an evidence-based algorithm and scoring system that enables more careful selection of patients for protected PCI to improve clinical outcomes.

ACKNOWLEDGMENTS

This review was supported by the Deutsches Zentrum fuer Herz-Kreislauf-Forschung - German Centre for Cardiovascular Research (DZHK). The authors thank Hyoin Bai for her excellent technical assistance.

DISCLOSURE

The authors have nothing to disclose.

CONFLICT OF INTEREST

The authors declare that they have no potential conflict of interest.

REFERENCES

1. Venkitachalam L, Kip KE, Selzer F, et al. Twenty-year evolution of percutaneous coronary intervention and its impact on clinical outcomes: a report from the National Heart, Lung, and Blood Institute-sponsored, multicenter 1985-1986 PTCA and 1997-2006 Dynamic Registries. Circ Cardiovasc Interv 2009;2(1):6–13.
2. Waldo SW, Secemsky EA, O'Brien C, et al. Surgical ineligibility and mortality among patients with unprotected left main or multivessel coronary artery disease undergoing percutaneous coronary intervention. Circulation 2014;130(25):2295–301.
3. Rihal CS, Naidu SS, Givertz MM, et al. 2015 SCAI/ACC/HFSA/STS clinical expert consensus Statement on the Use of percutaneous mechanical circulatory support devices in Cardiovascular Care: Endorsed by the American Heart Assocation, the Cardiological Society of India, and Sociedad Latino Americana de Cardiologia Intervencion; Affirmation of Value by the Canadian Association of Interventional Cardiology-Association Canadienne de Cardiologie d'intervention. J Am Coll Cardiol 2015;65(19):e7–26.
4. Basir MB, Kapur NK, Patel K, et al. Improved outcomes associated with the use of shock protocols: updates from the national cardiogenic shock initiative. Catheter Cardiovasc Interv 2019;93(7):1173–83.
5. Ameloot K, Bastos MB, Daemen J, et al. New-generation mechanical circulatory support during high-risk PCI: a cross-sectional analysis. EuroIntervention 2019;15(5):427–33.
6. Mennuni MG, Pagnotta PA, Stefanini GG. Coronary stents: the impact of technological advances on clinical outcomes. Ann Biomed Eng 2016;44(2):488–96.
7. Vetrovec GW. Hemodynamic support devices for shock and high-risk PCI: when and which one. Curr Cardiol Rep 2017;19(10):100.
8. Velazquez EJ, Lee KL, Jones RH, et al. Coronary-artery bypass surgery in patients with ischemic cardiomyopathy. N Engl J Med 2016;374(16):1511–20.
9. Nayyar M, Donovan KM, Khouzam RN. When more is not better-appropriately excluding patients from mechanical circulatory support therapy. Ann Transl Med 2018;6(1):9.
10. Nellis SH, Liedtke AJ, Whitesell L. Small coronary vessel pressure and diameter in an intact beating rabbit heart using fixed-position and free-motion techniques. Circ Res 1981;49(2):342–53.
11. Ait Ichou J, Larivee N, Eisenberg MJ, et al. The effectiveness and safety of the Impella ventricular assist device for high-risk percutaneous coronary interventions: a systematic review. Catheter Cardiovasc Interv 2018;91(7):1250–60.
12. Drakos SG, Kfoury AG, Selzman CH, et al. Left ventricular assist device unloading effects on myocardial structure and function: current status of the field and call for action. Curr Opin Cardiol 2011;26(3):245–55.
13. Burkhoff D, Sayer G, Doshi D, et al. Hemodynamics of mechanical circulatory support. J Am Coll Cardiol 2015;66(23):2663–74.
14. Csepe TA, Kilic A. Advancements in mechanical circulatory support for patients in acute and chronic heart failure. J Thorac Dis 2017;9(10):4070–83.
15. Briguori C, Sarais C, Pagnotta P, et al. Elective versus provisional intra-aortic balloon pumping in high-risk percutaneous transluminal coronary angioplasty. Am Heart J 2003;145(4):700–7.
16. Papaioannou TG, Stefanadis C. Basic principles of the intraaortic balloon pump and mechanisms affecting its performance. ASAIO J 2005;51(3):296–300.

17. Basra SS, Loyalka P, Kar B. Current status of percutaneous ventricular assist devices for cardiogenic shock. Curr Opin Cardiol 2011;26(6):548–54.

18. Raess DH, Weber DM. Impella 2.5. J Cardiovasc Transl Res 2009;2(2):168–72.

19. Kapur NK, Paruchuri V, Urbano-Morales JA, et al. Mechanically unloading the left ventricle before coronary reperfusion reduces left ventricular wall stress and myocardial infarct size. Circulation 2013;128(4):328–36.

20. Koeckert MS, Jorde UP, Naka Y, et al. 5 for left ventricular unloading during venoarterial extracorporeal membrane oxygenation support. J Card Surg 2011;26(6):666–8.

21. Bavaria JE, Ratcliffe MB, Gupta KB, et al. Changes in left ventricular systolic wall stress during biventricular circulatory assistance. Ann Thorac Surg 1988;45(5):526–32.

22. Atkinson TM, Ohman EM, O'Neill WW, et al, Interventional Scientific Council of the American College of Cardiology. A practical approach to mechanical circulatory support in patients undergoing percutaneous coronary intervention: an interventional perspective. JACC Cardiovasc Interv 2016;9(9):871–83.

23. Shamekhi J, Putz A, Zimmer S, et al. Impact of hemodynamic support on outcome in patients undergoing high-risk percutaneous coronary intervention. Am J Cardiol 2019;124(1):20–30.

24. Becher T, Eder F, Baumann S, et al. Unprotected versus protected high-risk percutaneous coronary intervention with the Impella 2.5 in patients with multivessel disease and severely reduced left ventricular function. Medicine (Baltimore) 2018;97(43): e12665.

25. Perera D, Stables R, Clayton T, et al. Long-term mortality data from the balloon pump-assisted coronary intervention study (BCIS-1): a randomized, controlled trial of elective balloon counterpulsation during high-risk percutaneous coronary intervention. Circulation 2013;127(2):207–12.

26. Maini B, Naidu SS, Mulukutla S, et al. Real-world use of the Impella 2.5 circulatory support system in complex high-risk percutaneous coronary intervention: the USpella Registry. Catheter Cardiovasc Interv 2012;80(5):717–25.

27. O'Neill WW, Kleiman NS, Moses J, et al. A prospective, randomized clinical trial of hemodynamic support with Impella 2.5 versus intra-aortic balloon pump in patients undergoing high-risk percutaneous coronary intervention: the PROTECT II study. Circulation 2012;126(14):1717–27.

28. Roques F, Nashef SA, Michel P, et al. Risk factors and outcome in European cardiac surgery: analysis of the EuroSCORE multinational database of 19030 patients. Eur J Cardiothorac Surg 1999;15(6):816–22 [discussion: 822–3].

29. Shahian DM, Jacobs JP, Badhwar V, et al. The Society of Thoracic Surgeons 2018 adult cardiac surgery risk models: part 1-background, design considerations, and model development. Ann Thorac Surg 2018;105(5):1411–8.

30. O'Brien SM, Feng L, He X, et al. The Society of Thoracic Surgeons 2018 adult cardiac surgery risk models: part 2-statistical methods and results. Ann Thorac Surg 2018;105(5):1419–28.

31. Baumann S, Werner N, Ibrahim K, et al. Indication and short-term clinical outcomes of high-risk percutaneous coronary intervention with microaxial Impella(R) pump: results from the German Impella(R) registry. Clin Res Cardiol 2018;107(8):653–7.

32. Kovacic JC, Nguyen HT, Karajgikar R, et al. The Impella Recover 2.5 and TandemHeart ventricular assist devices are safe and associated with equivalent clinical outcomes in patients undergoing high-risk percutaneous coronary intervention. Catheter Cardiovasc Interv 2013;82(1):E28–37.

33. Baumann S, Werner N, Al-Rashid F, et al. Six months follow-up of protected high-risk percutaneous coronary intervention with the microaxial Impella pump: results from the German Impella registry. Coron Artery Dis 2020;31(3):237–42.

34. Thiele H, Sick P, Boudriot E, et al. Randomized comparison of intra-aortic balloon support with a percutaneous left ventricular assist device in patients with revascularized acute myocardial infarction complicated by cardiogenic shock. Eur Heart J 2005;26(13):1276–83.

35. Lauten A, Engstrom AE, Jung C, et al. Percutaneous left-ventricular support with the Impella-2.5-assist device in acute cardiogenic shock: results of the Impella-EUROSHOCK-registry. Circ Heart Fail 2013;6(1):23–30.

36. Thiele H, Zeymer U, Neumann FJ, et al. Intraaortic balloon support for myocardial infarction with cardiogenic shock. N Engl J Med 2012;367(14): 1287–96.

37. Thiele H, Zeymer U, Neumann FJ, et al. Intra-aortic balloon counterpulsation in acute myocardial infarction complicated by cardiogenic shock (IABP-SHOCK II): final 12 month results of a randomised, open-label trial. Lancet 2013;382(9905): 1638–45.

38. Thiele H, Zeymer U, Thelemann N, et al. Intraaortic balloon pump in cardiogenic shock complicating acute myocardial infarction: long-term 6-year outcome of the randomized IABP-SHOCK II Trial. Circulation 2018. https://doi.org/10.1161/CIRCULATIONAHA.118.038201.

39. Myat A, Patel N, Tehrani S, et al. Percutaneous circulatory assist devices for high-risk coronary intervention. JACC Cardiovasc Interv 2015;8(2):229–44.

40. Rastan AJ, Tillmann E, Subramanian S, et al. Visceral arterial compromise during intra-aortic

balloon counterpulsation therapy. Circulation 2010;
122(11 Suppl):S92–9.

41. Asleh R, Resar JR. Utilization of percutaneous mechanical circulatory support devices in cardiogenic shock complicating acute myocardial infarction and high-risk percutaneous coronary interventions. J Clin Med 2019;8(8):1209.

42. Kar B, Basra SS, Shah NR, et al. Percutaneous circulatory support in cardiogenic shock: interventional bridge to recovery. Circulation 2012;125(14):1809–17.

43. Pham DT, Al-Quthami A, Kapur NK. Percutaneous left ventricular support in cardiogenic shock and severe aortic regurgitation. Catheter Cardiovasc Interv 2013;81(2):399–401.

44. Burzotta F, Trani C, Doshi SN, et al. Impella ventricular support in clinical practice: collaborative viewpoint from a European expert user group. Int J Cardiol 2015;201:684–91.

45. Pieri M, Agracheva N, Bonaveglio E, et al. Bivalirudin versus heparin as an anticoagulant during extracorporeal membrane oxygenation: a case-control study. J Cardiothorac Vasc Anesth 2013; 27(1):30–4.

46. Ibanez B, James S, Agewall S, et al. 2017 ESC guidelines for the management of acute myocardial infarction in patients presenting with ST-segment elevation. Rev Esp Cardiol (Engl Ed) 2017;70(12):1082.

47. Levine GN, Bates ER, Blankenship JC, et al. 2011 ACCF/AHA/SCAI guideline for percutaneous coronary intervention. A report of the American College of Cardiology Foundation/American Heart Association Task Force on practice guidelines and the Society for Cardiovascular Angiography and Interventions. J Am Coll Cardiol 2011;58(24):e44–122.

48. Werner N, Akin I, Al-Rashid F, et al. Expertenkonsensus zum praktischen Einsatz von Herzkreislaufunterstützungssystemen bei Hochrisiko-Koronarinterventionen. Kardiologe 2017;11:460–72.

49. McCabe JM. Hemodynamic support for CTO PCI: who, when & how. Presented at Transcatheter Cardiovascular Therapeutics (TCT). San Diego, CA, September 21–25, 2018.

Stent Thrombosis After Percutaneous Coronary Intervention

From Bare-Metal to the Last Generation of Drug-Eluting Stents

Alberto Polimeni, MD, PhD[a,b,1],
Sabato Sorrentino, MD, PhD[a,b,1],
Carmen Spaccarotella, MD[a,b],
Annalisa Mongiardo, MD[a],
Jolanda Sabatino, MD, PhD[a,b],
Salvatore De Rosa, MD, PhD[a,b], Tommaso Gori, MD, PhD[c],
Ciro Indolfi, MD[a,b,d,*]

KEYWORDS

- BMS • DES • BRS • Thrombosis • Stent

KEY POINTS

- Although rare, thrombosis still remains a major complication after coronary stent implantation.
- Although the causes of stent thrombosis are multifactorial, the device-related mechanism is a key factor.
- Knowing the different characteristics of the stents is of paramount importance for choosing the most suitable stent for the specific patient in clinical practice.

INTRODUCTION

The introduction in clinical practice of coronary stents has set a milestone in the history of interventional cardiology. Developed to overcome the limitation of plain old balloon angioplasty (POBA), this technology over the years has become a standard of care in the treatment of coronary artery disease. The continuous technical evolution has brought several types of stents to cope with the increasing complexity of the lesions that currently are accessible to the percutaneous approach. Accordingly, being familiar with the technical features of each platform and its related safety and efficacy profile is becoming of paramount importance. Stent thrombosis (ST) is an uncommon but harmful complication of percutaneous coronary implantation (PCI), causing myocardial infarction in

This article originally appeared in Cardiology Clinics, Volume 38, Issue 4, November 2020.
Conflict of interest statement: The authors have no conflicts of interest to declare.
[a] Division of Cardiology, Department of Medical and Surgical Sciences, "Magna Graecia" University, Viale Europa, Catanzaro 88100, Italy; [b] Research Center for Cardiovascular Diseases, "Magna Graecia" University, Viale Europa, Catanzaro 88100, Italy; [c] Kardiologie I, Zentrum für Kardiologie, University Medical Center Mainz, Deutsches Zentrum für Herz und Kreislauf Forschung, Langenbeckstraße 1, Standort Rhein-Main 55131, Germany; [d] Mediterranea Cardiocentro, Via Orazio, 2, Naples 80122, Italy
[1] These authors contributed equally to this work.
* Corresponding author. Division of Cardiology, Department of Medical and Surgical Sciences, "Magna Graecia" University, Viale Europa, Catanzaro 88100, Italy.
E-mail address: indolfi@unicz.it

Intervent Cardiol Clin 11 (2022) 465–473
https://doi.org/10.1016/j.iccl.2022.07.002

approximately 60% to 70% of the cases, and leading to an increased risk of mortality (20%–25%).[1] The type of stent implanted is a major factor in determining the risk of coronary ST.[2] Therefore, this review article describes evidence from clinical trials or observational studies on the coronary stent types used most often (Fig. 1) and their related risk of ST in the modern era of interventional cardiology.

BARE-METAL STENT

Bare-metal stents (BMSs) have been developed to avoid elastic recoil and late vascular remodeling after POBA. Since their introduction in clinical practice in 1986 with the Wallstent (Schneider AG) and in 1987 with the first Food and Drug Administration–approved Palmaz-Schatz stent (Johnson & Johnson), BMSs progressively replaced POBA and became standard of care for PCI in the late 1990s. Despite the continuous improvement in stent technology, however, long-term follow-up revealed 20% to 30% incidence of in-stent restenosis (ISR).[3] The high rate of ISR observed with these platforms is caused by the proliferation and migration of vascular smooth muscle cells within stent struts, a phenomenon widely studied using in vitro and in vivo models.[4–7] The introduction in clinical practice of drug-eluting stents (DESs) to overcome this limitation led to progressive decline in the use of BMSs, with a significant reduction of ISR. Several studies and registries have shown that the rates of early ST between BMSs and first-generation DESs were quite similar[8]; the risk of very late ST (VLST) was surprisingly higher with DESs, thus becoming a concern for fast and generalized use of medicated platforms.[9] Characteristics and potential mechanisms underlying VLST differ significantly between BMS and DES platforms. In 61 patients with VLST, reported by Nakamura and colleagues,[10] using the optical

coherence technique, the malapposed or uncovered strut and stent underexpansion were observed more frequently in DESs, whereas thin-cap fibroatheroma, neoatherosclerosis, and lipid neointima were observed more frequently in BMSs than in DESs.

Despite the improvement of implantation techniques and the introduction in clinical practice of the less thrombogenic second-generation DESs that ensure reasonable discontinuation of the dual antiplatelet therapy (DAPT),[11] the BMS has continued to be used for a long time, for those patients in whom a prolonged antithrombotic therapy did not ensure a reasonable risk-benefit tradeoff. The recently published Italian Multicenter Registry of Bare Metal Stent Use in Modern Percutaneous Coronary Intervention Era (AMARCORD) registry, including 58,879 patients undergoing PCI and stent implantation in 18 Italian sites, reported a progressive decrease in BMS use, from 10.1% in 2013% to 0.3%, in 2017. The main reasons for BMS implantation were ST-elevation myocardial infarction (STEMI) (23.1%), advanced age (24.4%), and physician perception of high bleeding risk (HBR) (34.0%). At a mean follow-up of 2.2 years ± 1.5 years, the rates of definitive ST were 2.3% (1.2% at 30 days and 1.9% at 1 year).[12] Several clinical trials and prospective studies have shown superiority of second-generation DESs compared with BMSs.

DURABLE POLYMER DRUG-ELUTING STENT

Evidence from post mortem pathology and intracoronary imaging supports the concept that the increased thrombosis observed in patients receiving first-generation DESs essentially was due to the fact that the cytotoxic drugs eluted by the stents inhibit not only the proliferation and migration of the vascular smooth

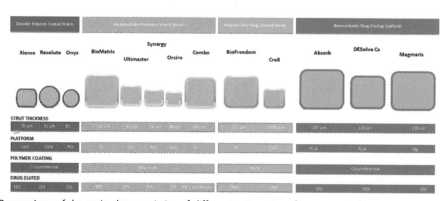

Fig. 1. Comparison of the main characteristics of different categories of coronary stent.

muscle cells that are responsible for restenosis but also the growth and mobility of endothelial cells, fundamental for the healing of the vessel after the stent implantation.[13,14] Furthermore, first-generation DESs were coated with permanent polymers like methacrylate compounds that facilitate drug release but remain on the stent after drug elution, causing vascular inflammation, hypereosinophilia, and thrombogenic reactions.[15,16] The increased stent strut thickness that was necessary to warrant sufficient radial strength to first-generation DESs also has a major impact in thrombosis. Several studies demonstrated that thick-strutted stents are more thrombogenic than comparable thin-strutted devices.[17]

The second-generation DESs were designed to overcome these safety issues, employing new and more biocompatible polymer coatings, less toxic antiproliferative drugs and thin-strut metal alloys. The introduction of cobalt chromium (CoCr), a more biocompatible material, increasingly is used in new-generation coronary stents. In comparison with stainless steel, CoCr has a higher radiopacity and radial strength. This allows for the production of thinner struts with a similar radiological visibility and radial strength. For all these reasons, the zotarolimus-eluting stent (ZES) and everolimus-eluting stent (EES) have demonstrated a decreased risk of late ST and very-late ST in comparison with old-generation DESs.

In the COMPARE trial, the rates of definite and probable ST were reduced significantly among EES compared with paclitaxel-eluting stent-treated patients (0.7% vs 2.6%, respectively; $P = .002$) at 12 months.[18] In recent work published by Tada and colleagues,[19] in unselected patients in a large German cohort, the cumulative incidence of definite ST at 3 years was 1.5% with the BMS, 2.2% with the first-generation DESs, and 1.0% with the second-generation DESs. The consistent superiority of newer-generation DESs also is demonstrated in meta-analyses, showing odds ratios between 0.31 and 0.56 for ST in different DES types compared with BMSs.[20] Furthermore, much evidence also supports second-generation DESs for those patients who historically have been treated with BMSs, because of low risk of ISR or high risk of early coronary thrombotic events (such as STEMI patients) or because of not tolerating a prolonged DAPT (such as HBR patients). In regard to STEMI patients, several clinical trials and observational registries have shown superiority of DESs over BMSs.[21,22] In a large pooled analysis, including 2665 patients enrolled in the Clinical Evaluation of the Xience-V stent in Acute Myocardial Infarction) (EXAMINATION) and Comparison of Biolimus Eluted From an Erodible Stent Coating With Bare Metal Stents in Acute ST-Elevation Myocardial Infarction (COMFORTABLE-AMI) trials, newer-generation DESs were associated with a significant reduction of 1-year definite ST (relative risk 0.35; 95% CI, 0.16–0.75; $P = .006$) compared with BMSs.[22]

For patients with large vessel diameter, BMSs seemed a reasonable option, because of the theoretically lower risk of developing a clinical overt ISR. Despite a similar risk of ST compared with DESs, BMSs have shown higher rates of stent failure. In a recently published post hoc analysis from the EXAMINATION trial, including 1498 patients with ST-segment elevated myocardial infarction undergoing primary PCI, despite no differences in terms of ST between groups, DES implantation was associated with a trend toward a reduction of the target lesion (hazard ratio [HR] 0.53; 95% CI, 0.27–1.02; $P = .05$) and target vessel revascularization (HR 0.60; 95% CI, 0.34–1.03; $P = .066$) in patients with larger vessel diameter.[23]

Finally, the perception of HBR has become the most frequent reason supporting BMS implantation in these last years. The rationale underlying this choice is the possibility of avoiding the prolonged antithrombotic therapy required to prevent the mild and long-term risk of ST observed with DESs.[24–27] Improvement in stent technology and implantation technique, however, significantly decreased such risk, thus supporting early DAPT discontinuation after DES implantation even for this subgroup of patients.[25] Several trials and prospective registries have shown the superiority of the second-generation DESs over BMSs under a mandated short DAPT period.[28,29]

Recently, the ZEUS study[30] showed that a treatment strategy consisting of ZES implantation followed by a personalized course of DAPT, resulted in a lower risk of major adverse cardiac events (MACEs) and definite or probable ST compared with BMSs (ST, 2.0% vs 4.1%, respectively; $P = .019$) in patients at HBR or thrombosis or at low risk of restenosis (no planned stent <3.0 mm diameter was intended to be implanted) at 1-year follow-up. Several studies recently have been published, or are ongoing, aiming at generalizing this concept to an even more larger types of DESs in HBR population, including the Xience Short DAPT programs (NCT03218787), the EVOLVE Short DAPT[31] (NCT02605447), the ONYX ONE[32] (NCT03344653), the POEM (NCT03112707), and MASTER DAPT[33] (NCT03023020) studies. The ONYX trial, randomizing either Resolute Onyx (Medtronic, CA, USA) DES (durable polymer [DP] DES) (n = 1003) or BioFreedom polymer-free [PF]-drug-coated stent (DCS) (n = 993) with 1-month DAPT, documented noninferiority of the DP-ZES compared with the Bio-Freedom DCS in the primary endpoint, including death from cardiac causes, myocardial infarction, or ST, with no differences in the rate of ST between groups (1.3% for the Onyx DES and 2.1% for the BMS).

Looking at the long-term performances of second-generation DESs in this high-risk population, in a pooled analysis from 4 all-comer post-approval registries that included 10,502 HBR patients who underwent PCI with CoCr-EES implantation, the 4-year rate of probable or definite ST was 1.5%.[34] Rates were similar to the ones observed in other all-comers registries testing the long-term effectiveness of CoCr-EES. For example, the Randomized Comparison of a Zotarolimus-Eluting Stent With an Everolimus-Eluting Stent for Percutaneous Coronary Intervention (RESOLUTE) trial, randomizing patients to Resolute ZES (R-ZES) (n = 1140) or CoCr-EES (n = 1152), showed 1.6% and 2.3% of ST at 4 years of follow-up, respectively, in the EES and R-ZES groups.

BIORESORBABLE POLYMER DRUG-ELUTING STENT

Another direction to improve drug-carrier systems was the development of erodible polymers. Biodegradable polymers (BPs) remain temporary on the DES surface and have the potential to enhance biocompatibility and improve the delayed healing in the vessel. These stents use BPs that remain only temporarily on the DES surface and have the potential of less chronic vessel wall inflammation, similar to a BMS, as reported by Yin and colleagues.[35]

Long-term data, however, after implantation of newer generations of thin-strut BP-based DESs still are lacking. A meta-analysis by Cassese and colleagues[36] showed for the first time that the ultra–thin-strut BP–sirolimus-eluting stent (SES) displays a performance comparable to the DP-EES, the benchmark of contemporary DESs, also for ST (1.3% vs 1.9%; P = .45) at 1-year follow-up, and, more interestingly, there was no time-dependent risk of ST associated with BP-SES versus DP-EES.

Long-term data are available only for early-generation BP–biolimus eluting-stents (BESs). Lu and colleagues[37] showed that BP-BESs were associated with lower rates of MACEs, target lesion revascularization, and ST (2.6% vs 3.8%, respectively; P = .003) to the DP-DES of first and second generations at 5 years of follow-up. When BP-BES was compared with CoCr-EES, however, no differences in ST (BP-BES 0.4% vs CoCr-EES 0.7%) were observed at 2-year follow-up[38] and also at longer-term follow-up (5 years).[39] With the intention of improving the characteristics of the BP-DES, in terms of strut thickness, polymer biodegradation coating, and drug release kinetics, new devices were developed. The Synergy (Boston Scientific, Marlborough, USA) BP-DES, a novel thin-strut platinum/chromium alloy stent that elutes everolimus from a rapid BP matrix, was one of the most intensively studied. In the EVOLVE II trial, it was noninferior to the PROMUS (Boston Scientific, Marlborough, USA) Element Plus EES with respect to definite/probable ST (0.4% vs 0.6%, respectively; P = .50) at 1-year follow-up.[40]

The Orsiro coronary stent (Biotronik AG, Bülach, Switzerland) consists of an ultra–thin-strut CoCr design with a bioresorbable, poly-L lactic acid polymer coating that elutes the antiproliferative drug sirolimus. This bioresorbable polymer SES was evaluated in the BIOFLOW V trial. At 1-year follow-up, the number of patients with late ST was significantly lower in the bioresorbable polymer SES group than in the DP-EES group, despite similar rates of definite or probable ST between groups (<1% vs 1%, respectively; P = .694).[41]

POLYMER-FREE DRUG-ELUTING STENT

To overcome the limitations related to DPs and BPs, PF-DES platforms were introduced. Elimination of the polymer might lower the rates of late ST, as suggested by previous studies in comparison with first-generation DESs.[42] The attainment of optimal drug-release kinetics, however, is the real challenge of PF-DES technology. First-generation devices had the limit of a too rapid drug elution (90% within 2 days) and failed to achieve the desirable inhibition of neointima formation.[43] After that, several randomized controlled trials were performed to evaluate the clinical performance of different PF-DES platforms. Recently, the MiStent, a DES with a fully absorbable polymer coating containing and embedding a microcrystalline form of sirolimus into the vessel wall, was evaluated in the DES-SOLVE III trial[44] At 1-year follow-up, the rate of definite/probable ST was similar in comparison with DP-EES (0.7% vs 0.9%, respectively; P = .76).

Despite their improvements, PF platforms showed clinical outcomes and rates of ST comparable with modern permanent or BP-based DES up to 5 years' follow-up[45] Recently, Torii and colleagues[46] tested the hypothesis that the fluoropolymer on EES (FP-EES) is the most important component of its design with respect to thromboresistance by comparing stents of similar design with and without coating in a swine ex vivo shunt model. They demonstrated that FP-EES has the lowest platelet adherence compared with BP-DES, PF-DES, and BMS, with the lowest inflammatory cell density. These results reflect the phenomenon of fluoropassivation, representing one proposed mechanism for clinically observed low ST rates in FP-EES.[46] Because of their supposed lower risk of VLST, PF-DESs have been tested in high-risk profile populations, such as patients at HBR or with diabetes. The LEADERS FREE trial randomized 2466 HBR patients to either the BioFreedom DCS (Biosensors Europe, Morges, Switzerland) or a similar BMS undergoing PCI under a 1-month mandated DAPT therapy. DESs were noted to be superior to BMSs for the primary composite endpoint, including cardiac death, MI, or ST at 2 years of follow-up, with a similar 2-year rate of definite/probable ST between the groups (2.1% for the DCS and 2.3% for the BMS). The Cre8 stent (CID SpA, member of Alvimedica, Saluggia, Italy) is an 80-μm–strut thickness CoCr PF-DES, releasing sirolimus from reservoirs placed on the abluminal stent surface. In a recently published propensity match analysis pooling 2 recent multicenter, observational independent studies conducted at 22 Italian centers, such as the Amphilimus Italian Multicentre Registry (ASTUTE) and the Polymer Free Biolimus-Eluting Stent Implantation in All-Comers Population (RUDI-FREE), aimed at comparing the safety and efficacy profile of Cre8 stent and Bio-Freedom biolimus-eluting stent (BES) PF-DESs in real-world patients undergoing PCI. In a total population of 2320 patients, both BES and Cre8 stents had similar rates of 1-year target lesion failure (4.2% vs 4.0%, respectively; HR 0.98; 95% CI; 0.57–1.70) as well as low 1-year rate of definite or probable ST (0.9% and 0.8%, respectively; HR 1.17; 95% CI, 0.36–3.81). The subgroup analysis showed a potential benefit of Cre8 in patients with diabetes mellitus, while of BioFreedom BES in patients without diabetes mellitus (P for interaction = 0.002).[47] Randomized trials comparing PF-DES to the DP-DES, however, are warranted to establish the safety and efficacy profile of these platforms in dedicated subgroups of patients.

BIORESORBABLE VASCULAR SCAFFOLD

In order to overcome the limits of DESs, fully bioresorbable scaffolds (BRSs) were introduced in 2012. The most studied BRS was the Absorb BVS.[48] Despite promising results at short-term follow-up, the Absorb BVS showed an increase of in-scaffold thrombosis in comparison with EES at long-term follow-up.[49–53]

The negative results of ABSORB II and AIDA at 3 years' follow-up[54,55] confirmed by several meta-analyses (ST, BRS 2.4% vs EES 0.7%),[52,56–59] resulted in the end of Absorb BVS use and withdrawal from the market in September 2017.

The experience with Absorb BVS, however, provided some precious lessons, in particular about the paramount role of implantation techniques. Several studies[60–65] in different clinical settings showed that an optimal deployment technique—pre-dilation, proper sizing, and post-dilation[66,67]—significantly reduced the rates of scaffold thrombosis (ScT), the Achilles heel of Absorb BVS.[68] These results were contrasted across the studies and some doubt remained whether the risk of ScT is due to the Absorb BVS platform or the implantation technique.[69]

The initial assumption of BRSs was to provide temporary mechanical support to the vessel without compromising the restoration of vascular physiology with the potential of preventing late adverse events after the complete resorption.[70] The 5-year outcome data of ABSORB Japan[71] showed that there were no significant differences in the composite or individual endpoint outcomes between the Absorb BVS and Xience arms through 5 years or between 3 years and 5 years. Similar results were reported in a single-center study, where the incidence of very late adverse events in patients with a BRS implantation decreased over years (ScT was 3.6% in the first year, 2.2% in the second-third year, and 0.6% in the fourth to fifth years after implantation). Recently, a summary-level meta-analysis by Stone and colleagues[72] of 4 trials, reporting 5-year follow-up data, showed a ScT in 0.1% of BVS-treated patients versus 0.3% of EES-treated patients between 3 years and 5 years (HR 0.44; 95% CI, 0.07–2.70) (P for interaction = .03), suggesting that the period of ScT risk for the Absorb BVS ends at 3 years.

OTHER BIORESORBABLE PLATFORMS

In such a scenario, the Biotronik magnesium-based Magmaris, Fantom (Reva Medical, San

Diego, California), poly-L lactide-based polymer scaffold (Elixir Medical Corporation, Sunnyvale, California), ART (Terumo, Tokyo, Japan), and several other ones, including materials, such as tyrosine polycarbonate, salicylic acid polymer, and iron, were introduced. Although promising, the use of these devices in clinical practice is currently limited for the lack of randomized clinical studies and the current guidelines that limit their use.[73]

Recently, despite initial success of first studies, the Reva Medical company filed for bankruptcy protection in early 2020, although the next-generation DREAMS 3G, the evolution of Magmaris, with thinner struts and prolonged scaffolding time while keeping a 12-month resorption time, is being tested in the First in Men Study (BIOMAG-I; NCT04157153) and will be available for clinical trials in the near future.

Finally, it is unclear if the material technology will allow in future to overcome the limitations of current BRSs.

REFERENCES

1. Cutlip DE, Baim DS, Ho KK, et al. Stent thrombosis in the modern era: a pooled analysis of multicenter coronary stent clinical trials. Circulation 2001; 103(15):1967–71.
2. D'Ascenzo F, Iannaccone M, Saint-Hilary G, et al. Impact of design of coronary stents and length of dual antiplatelet therapies on ischaemic and bleeding events: a network meta-analysis of 64 randomized controlled trials and 102 735 patients. Eur Heart J 2017;38(42):3160–72.
3. Kastrati A, Mehilli J, Pache J, et al. Analysis of 14 trials comparing sirolimus-eluting stents with bare-metal stents. N Engl J Med 2007;356(10):1030–9.
4. Iaconetti C, Polimeni A, Sorrentino S, et al. Inhibition of miR-92a increases endothelial proliferation and migration in vitro as well as reduces neointimal proliferation in vivo after vascular injury. Basic Res Cardiol 2012;107(5):296.
5. Iaconetti C, De Rosa S, Polimeni A, et al. Downregulation of miR-23b induces phenotypic switching of vascular smooth muscle cells in vitro and in vivo. Cardiovasc Res 2015;107(4):522–33.
6. Gareri C, Iaconetti C, Sorrentino S, et al. miR-125a-5p modulates phenotypic switch of vascular smooth muscle cells by targeting ETS-1. J Mol Biol 2017;429(12):1817–28.
7. Sorrentino S, Iaconetti C, De Rosa S, et al. Hindlimb ischemia impairs endothelial recovery and increases neointimal proliferation in the carotid artery. Sci Rep 2018;8(1):761.
8. Roukoz H, Bavry AA, Sarkees ML, et al. Comprehensive meta-analysis on drug-eluting stents versus bare-metal stents during extended follow-up. Am J Med 2009;122(6):581 e581–510.
9. Camenzind E, Steg PG, Wijns W. Stent thrombosis late after implantation of first-generation drug-eluting stents: a cause for concern. Circulation 2007;115(11):1440–55 [discussion: 1455].
10. Nakamura D, Attizzani GF, Toma C, et al. Failure mechanisms and neoatherosclerosis patterns in very late drug-eluting and bare-metal stent thrombosis. Circ Cardiovasc Interv 2016;9(9):e003785.
11. Sorrentino S, Giustino G, Baber U, et al. Dual antiplatelet therapy cessation and adverse events after drug-eluting stent implantation in patients at high risk for atherothrombosis (from the PARIS Registry). Am J Cardiol 2018;122(10):1638–46.
12. Giannini F, Pagnesi M, Campo G, et al. Italian multicenter registry of bare metal stent use in modern percutaneous coronary intervention era (AMARCORD): a multicenter observational study. Catheter Cardiovasc Interv 2020. https://doi.org/10.1002/ccd.28798.
13. Curcio A, Torella D, Cuda G, et al. Effect of stent coating alone on in vitro vascular smooth muscle cell proliferation and apoptosis. Am J Physiol Heart Circ Physiol 2004;286(3):H902–8.
14. Joner M, Finn AV, Farb A, et al. Pathology of drug-eluting stents in humans: delayed healing and late thrombotic risk. J Am Coll Cardiol 2006;48(1):193–202.
15. Virmani R, Guagliumi G, Farb A, et al. Localized hypersensitivity and late coronary thrombosis secondary to a sirolimus-eluting stent: should we be cautious? Circulation 2004;109(6):701–5.
16. Virmani R, Liistro F, Stankovic G, et al. Mechanism of late in-stent restenosis after implantation of a paclitaxel derivate-eluting polymer stent system in humans. Circulation 2002;106(21):2649–51.
17. Kolandaivelu K, Swaminathan R, Gibson WJ, et al. Stent thrombogenicity early in high-risk interventional settings is driven by stent design and deployment and protected by polymer-drug coatings. Circulation 2011;123(13):1400–9.
18. Kedhi E, Joesoef KS, McFadden E, et al. Second-generation everolimus-eluting and paclitaxel-eluting stents in real-life practice (COMPARE): a randomised trial. Lancet 2010;375(9710):201–9.
19. Tada T, Byrne RA, Simunovic I, et al. Risk of stent thrombosis among bare-metal stents, first-generation drug-eluting stents, and second-generation drug-eluting stents: results from a registry of 18,334 patients. JACC Cardiovasc Interv 2013; 6(12):1267–74.
20. Kang SH, Park KW, Kang DY, et al. Biodegradable-polymer drug-eluting stents vs. bare metal stents vs. durable-polymer drug-eluting stents: a systematic review and Bayesian approach network meta-analysis. Eur Heart J 2014;35(17):1147–58.

21. Raber L, Kelbaek H, Ostojic M, et al. Effect of biolimus-eluting stents with biodegradable polymer vs bare-metal stents on cardiovascular events among patients with acute myocardial infarction: the COMFORTABLE AMI randomized trial. JAMA 2012;308(8):777–87.

22. Sabate M, Raber L, Heg D, et al. Comparison of newer-generation drug-eluting with bare-metal stents in patients with acute ST-segment elevation myocardial infarction: a pooled analysis of the EX-AMINATION (clinical evaluation of the Xience-V stent in acute myocardial INfArcTION) and COMFORTABLE-AMI (comparison of biolimus eluted from an erodible stent coating with bare metal stents in acute ST-elevation myocardial infarction) trials. JACC Cardiovasc Interv 2014;7(1): 55–63.

23. Costa F, Brugaletta S, Pernigotti A, et al. Does large vessel size justify use of bare-metal stents in primary percutaneous coronary intervention? Circ Cardiovasc Interv 2019;12(9):e007705.

24. Sorrentino S, Baber U, Claessen BE, et al. Determinants of significant out-of-hospital bleeding in patients undergoing percutaneous coronary intervention. Thromb Haemost 2018;118(11):1997–2005.

25. Sorrentino S, Sartori S, Baber U, et al. Bleeding risk, dual antiplatelet therapy cessation, and adverse events after percutaneous coronary intervention: the PARIS registry. Circ Cardiovasc Interv 2020; 13(4):e008226.

26. Faggioni M, Baber U, Sartori S, et al. Influence of baseline anemia on dual antiplatelet therapy cessation and risk of adverse events after percutaneous coronary intervention. Circ Cardiovasc Interv 2019; 12(4):e007133.

27. Schoos M, Chandrasekhar J, Baber U, et al. Causes, timing, and impact of dual antiplatelet therapy interruption for surgery (from the patterns of non-adherence to anti-platelet regimens in stented patients registry). Am J Cardiol 2017;120(6):904–10.

28. Ariotti S, Adamo M, Costa F, et al. Is bare-metal stent implantation still justifiable in high bleeding risk patients undergoing percutaneous coronary intervention?: a pre-specified analysis from the zeus trial. JACC Cardiovasc Interv 2016;9(5):426–36.

29. Urban P, Meredith IT, Abizaid A, et al. Polymer-free drug-coated coronary stents in patients at high bleeding risk. N Engl J Med 2015;373(21):2038–47.

30. Valgimigli M, Patialiakas A, Thury A, et al. Zotarolimus-eluting versus bare-metal stents in uncertain drug-eluting stent candidates. J Am Coll Cardiol 2015;65(8):805–15.

31. Mauri L, Kirtane AJ, Windecker S, et al. Rationale and design of the EVOLVE Short DAPT Study to assess 3-month dual antiplatelet therapy in subjects at high risk for bleeding undergoing percutaneous coronary intervention. Am Heart J 2018;205:110–7.

32. Kedhi E, Latib A, Abizaid A, et al. Rationale and design of the Onyx ONE global randomized trial: a randomized controlled trial of high-bleeding risk patients after stent placement with 1month of dual antiplatelet therapy. Am Heart J 2019;214: 134–41.

33. Frigoli E, Smits P, Vranckx P, et al. Design and rationale of the management of high bleeding risk patients post bioresorbable polymer coated stent implantation with an abbreviated versus standard DAPT regimen (MASTER DAPT) study. Am Heart J 2019;209:97–105.

34. Sorrentino S, Claessen BE, Chandiramani R, et al. Long-term safety and efficacy of durable polymer cobalt-chromium everolimus-eluting stents in patients at high bleeding risk: a patient-level stratified analysis from four postapproval studies. Circulation 2020;141(11):891–901.

35. Yin Y, Zhang Y, Zhao X. Safety and efficacy of biodegradable drug-eluting vs. bare metal stents: a meta-analysis from randomized trials. PLoS One 2014;9(6):e99648.

36. Cassese S, Ndrepepa G, Byrne RA, et al. Outcomes of patients treated with ultrathin strut biodegradable-polymer sirolimus-eluting stents versus fluoropolymer-based everolimus-eluting stents. A meta-analysis of randomized trials. Euro-Intervention 2018;14(2):224–31.

37. Lu P, Lu S, Li Y, et al. A comparison of the main outcomes from BP-BES and DP-DES at five years of follow-up: a systematic review and meta-analysis. Sci Rep 2017;7(1):14997.

38. Kaiser C, Galatius S, Jeger R, et al. Long-term efficacy and safety of biodegradable-polymer biolimus-eluting stents: main results of the Basel Stent Kosten-Effektivitats Trial-PROspective Validation Examination II (BASKET-PROVE II), a randomized, controlled noninferiority 2-year outcome trial. Circulation 2015;131(1):74–81.

39. Vlachojannis GJ, Smits PC, Hofma SH, et al. Biodegradable polymer biolimus-eluting stents versus durable polymer everolimus-eluting stents in patients with coronary artery disease: Final 5-year report from the COMPARE II trial (abluminal biodegradable polymer biolimus-eluting stent versus durable polymer everolimus-eluting stent). JACC Cardiovasc Interv 2017;10(12):1215–21.

40. Kereiakes DJ, Meredith IT, Windecker S, et al. Efficacy and safety of a novel bioabsorbable polymer-coated, everolimus-eluting coronary stent: the EVOLVE II randomized trial. Circ Cardiovasc Interv 2015;8(4):e002372.

41. Kandzari DE, Mauri L, Koolen JJ, et al. Ultrathin, bioresorbable polymer sirolimus-eluting stents versus thin, durable polymer everolimus-eluting

stents in patients undergoing coronary revascularisation (BIOFLOW V): a randomised trial. Lancet 2017;390(10105):1843–52.

42. Urban P, Macaya C, Rupprecht HJ, et al. Randomized evaluation of anticoagulation versus antiplatelet therapy after coronary stent implantation in high-risk patients: the multicenter aspirin and ticlopidine trial after intracoronary stenting (MATTIS). Circulation 1998;98(20):2126–32.

43. Hausleiter J, Kastrati A, Wessely R, et al. Prevention of restenosis by a novel drug-eluting stent system with a dose-adjustable, polymer-free, on-site stent coating. Eur Heart J 2005;26(15):1475–81.

44. de Winter RJ, Katagiri Y, Asano T, et al. A sirolimus-eluting bioabsorbable polymer-coated stent (MiStent) versus an everolimus-eluting durable polymer stent (Xience) after percutaneous coronary intervention (DESSOLVE III): a randomised, single-blind, multicentre, non-inferiority, phase 3 trial. Lancet 2018;391(10119):431–40.

45. Gao K, Sun Y, Yang M, et al. Efficacy and safety of polymer-free stent versus polymer-permanent drug-eluting stent in patients with acute coronary syndrome: a meta-analysis of randomized control trials. BMC Cardiovasc Disord 2017;17(1):194.

46. Torii S, Cheng Q, Mori H, et al. Acute thrombogenicity of fluoropolymer-coated versus biodegradable and polymer free stents. EuroIntervention 2018;14(16):1685–93.

47. Chiarito M, Sardella G, Colombo A, et al. Safety and efficacy of polymer-free drug-eluting stents. Circ Cardiovasc Interv 2019;12(2):e007311.

48. Indolfi C, De Rosa S, Colombo A. Bioresorbable vascular scaffolds - basic concepts and clinical outcome. Nat Rev Cardiol 2016;13(12):719–29.

49. Ali ZA, Gao R, Kimura T, et al. Three-year outcomes with the absorb bioresorbable scaffold: individual-patient-data meta-analysis from the ABSORB randomized trials. Circulation 2018;137(5):464–79.

50. Ali ZA, Serruys PW, Kimura T, et al. 2-year outcomes with the Absorb bioresorbable scaffold for treatment of coronary artery disease: a systematic review and meta-analysis of seven randomised trials with an individual patient data substudy. Lancet 2017;390(10096):760–72.

51. Kereiakes DJ, Ellis SG, Metzger C, et al. 3-year clinical outcomes with everolimus-eluting bioresorbable coronary scaffolds: the ABSORB III trial. J Am Coll Cardiol 2017;70(23):2852–62.

52. Stone GW, Gao R, Kimura T, et al. 1-year outcomes with the Absorb bioresorbable scaffold in patients with coronary artery disease: a patient-level, pooled meta-analysis. Lancet 2016;387(10025):1277–89.

53. Chevalier B, Cequier A, Dudek D, et al. Four-year follow-up of the randomised comparison between an everolimus-eluting bioresorbable scaffold and an everolimus-eluting metallic stent for the treatment of coronary artery stenosis (ABSORB II Trial). EuroIntervention 2018;13(13):1561–4.

54. Serruys PW, Chevalier B, Sotomi Y, et al. Comparison of an everolimus-eluting bioresorbable scaffold with an everolimus-eluting metallic stent for the treatment of coronary artery stenosis (ABSORB II): a 3 year, randomised, controlled, single-blind, multicentre clinical trial. Lancet 2016;388(10059):2479–91.

55. Wykrzykowska JJ, Kraak RP, Hofma SH, et al. Bioresorbable scaffolds versus metallic stents in routine PCI. N Engl J Med 2017;376(24):2319–28.

56. Polimeni A, Anadol R, Munzel T, et al. Long-term outcome of bioresorbable vascular scaffolds for the treatment of coronary artery disease: a meta-analysis of RCTs. BMC Cardiovasc Disord 2017; 17(1):147.

57. Sorrentino S, Giustino G, Mehran R, et al. Everolimus-eluting bioresorbable scaffolds versus everolimus-eluting metallic stents. J Am Coll Cardiol 2017;69(25):3055–66.

58. Collet C, Asano T, Sotomi Y, et al. Early, late and very late incidence of bioresorbable scaffold thrombosis: a systematic review and meta-analysis of randomized clinical trials and observational studies. Minerva Cardioangiol 2017;65(1):32–51.

59. Mukete BN, van der Heijden LC, Tandjung K, et al. Safety and efficacy of everolimus-eluting bioresorbable vascular scaffolds versus durable polymer everolimus-eluting metallic stents assessed at 1-year follow-up: a systematic review and meta-analysis of studies. Int J Cardiol 2016;221:1087–94.

60. Polimeni A, Anadol R, Munzel T, et al. Bioresorbable vascular scaffolds for percutaneous treatment of chronic total coronary occlusions: a meta-analysis. BMC Cardiovasc Disord 2019;19(1): 59.

61. Polimeni A, Weissner M, Schochlow K, et al. Incidence, clinical presentation, and predictors of clinical restenosis in coronary bioresorbable scaffolds. JACC Cardiovasc Interv 2017;10(18):1819–27.

62. Anadol R, Lorenz L, Weissner M, et al. Characteristics and outcome of patients with complex coronary lesions treated with bioresorbable scaffolds: three-year follow-up in a cohort of consecutive patients. EuroIntervention 2018;14(9):e1011–9.

63. Anadol R, Dimitriadis Z, Polimeni A, et al. Bioresorbable everolimus-eluting vascular scaffold for patients presenting with non STelevation-acute coronary syndrome: a three-years follow-up1. Clin Hemorheol Microcirc 2018;69(1–2):3–8.

64. Anadol R, Schnitzler K, Lorenz L, et al. Three-years outcomes of diabetic patients treated with coronary bioresorbable scaffolds. BMC Cardiovasc Disord 2018;18(1):92.

65. Polimeni A, Anadol R, Munzel T, et al. Predictors of bioresorbable scaffold failure in STEMI patients at 3years follow-up. Int J Cardiol 2018;268:68–74.

66. Sorrentino S, De Rosa S, Ambrosio G, et al. The duration of balloon inflation affects the luminal diameter of coronary segments after bioresorbable vascular scaffolds deployment. BMC Cardiovasc Disord 2015;15:169.

67. Dimitriadis Z, Polimeni A, Anadol R, et al. Procedural predictors for bioresorbable vascular scaffold thrombosis: analysis of the individual components of the "PSP" technique. J Clin Med 2019;8(1):93.

68. Gori T, Weissner M, Gonner S, et al. Characteristics, predictors, and mechanisms of thrombosis in coronary bioresorbable scaffolds: differences between early and late events. JACC Cardiovasc Interv 2017;10(23):2363–71.

69. Polimeni A, Gori T. Bioresorbable vascular scaffold: a step back thinking of the future. Postepy Kardiol Interwencyjnej 2018;14(2):117–9.

70. Gori T, Polimeni A, Indolfi C, et al. Predictors of stent thrombosis and their implications for clinical practice. Nat Rev Cardiol 2019;16(4):243–56.

71. Kozuma K, Tanabe K, Hamazaki Y, et al. Long-term outcomes of absorb bioresorbable vascular scaffold vs. everolimus-eluting metallic stent- a randomized comparison through 5 years in Japan. Circ J 2020;84(5):733–41.

72. Stone GW, Kimura T, Gao R, et al. Time-varying outcomes with the absorb bioresorbable vascular scaffold during 5-year follow-up: a systematic meta-analysis and individual patient data pooled study. JAMA Cardiol 2019;4(12):1261–9.

73. Haude M, Ince H, Abizaid A, et al. Sustained safety and performance of the second-generation drug-eluting absorbable metal scaffold in patients with de novo coronary lesions: 12-month clinical results and angiographic findings of the BIOSOLVE-II first-in-man trial. Eur Heart J 2016; 37(35):2701–9.

Moving?

Make sure your subscription moves with you!

To notify us of your new address, find your **Clinics Account Number** (located on your mailing label above your name), and contact customer service at:

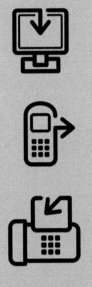

Email: journalscustomerservice-usa@elsevier.com

800-654-2452 (subscribers in the U.S. & Canada)
314-447-8871 (subscribers outside of the U.S. & Canada)

Fax number: 314-447-8029

Elsevier Health Sciences Division
Subscription Customer Service
3251 Riverport Lane
Maryland Heights, MO 63043

ELSEVIER